IMMUNE
SYSTEM
HACKS

175+ WAYS TO BOOST YOUR IMMUNITY, PROTECT AGAINST VIRUSES AND DISEASE, AND FEEL YOUR VERY BEST!

MATT FARR

Adams Media
New York   London   Toronto   Sydney   New Delhi

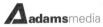

Adams Media
An Imprint of Simon & Schuster, Inc.
57 Littlefield Street
Avon, Massachusetts 02322

First Adams Media trade paperback edition December 2020

ADAMS MEDIA and colophon are trademarks of Simon & Schuster.

For information about special discounts for bulk purchases, please contact Simon & Schuster Special Sales at 1-866-506-1949 or business@simonandschuster.com.

The Simon & Schuster Speakers Bureau can bring authors to your live event. For more information or to book an event contact the Simon & Schuster Speakers Bureau at 1-866-248-3049 or visit our website at www.simonspeakers.com.

Manufactured in the United States of America

1 2020

Library of Congress Cataloging-in-Publication Data
Names: Farr, Matt, author.
Title: Immune system hacks / Matt Farr.
Description: Avon, Massachusetts: Adams Media, 2020. | Series: Hacks | Includes index.
Identifiers: LCCN 2020034711 | ISBN 9781507215258 (pb) | ISBN 9781507215265 (ebook)
Subjects: LCSH: Natural immunity. | Nutrition. | Immune system. | Self-care, Health.
Classification: LCC QR185.2 .F37 2020 | DDC 616.07/9--dc23
LC record available at https://lccn.loc.gov/2020034711

ISBN 978-1-5072-1525-8
ISBN 978-1-5072-1526-5 (ebook)

CONTENTS

INTRODUCTION

It's time to live your healthiest life!

The immune system is unique to any other system of your body as it has access to all your cells and tissues, working around the clock to protect you from germs, viruses, and more. It's deeply connected not just to every other system, but also to your environment and even your emotions. Everything from food sensitivity to stress can affect your immune health, and improving one means improving the other. To regulate your immune system is to regulate your whole being—body *and* mind.

But just how do you nurture a healthy immune system? *Immune System Hacks* is here to help you do just that! In this book, you'll find more than 175 easy hacks for developing a healthier, better functioning immune system. From foods and supplements that can protect against illness, to habits and therapies that heal chronic inflammation, there are hacks for almost every situation and immune condition. You'll discover holistic approaches to optimizing your immune system that also support your social, mental, emotional, and spiritual well-being.

Whether you are looking to protect yourself against infection, fight a current infection, reduce inflammation, or improve an allergy or auto-immune condition, this book will help you feel your best for years to come. Flip around to the hacks that stand out to you or read through each immune-boosting page.

MAKE FRIENDS WITH FUNGI

When choosing foods to help your immune system it's hard to beat mushrooms. Mushrooms contain beta-glucan, a fiber that, when consumed, challenges and stimulates a response within the immune system to increase white blood cells that help fight infections. Over time, this effect strengthens the immune system. Among other uses, beta-glucan's benefits have led to it being used in cancer therapy to help fight cancer cell growth.

In addition to boosting immunity, beta-glucan has also been shown to:

- Lower cholesterol
- Suppress appetite
- Slow the absorption of glucose from the gut into the bloodstream (benefiting those with insulin resistance/diabetes)

There are nutritional supplements available that contain beta-glucan, but you can also source it from your diet by consuming foods such as mushrooms, oats, and barley. The added benefit of consuming mushrooms specifically is that they also contain some of the highest levels of plant-based vitamin D, another immunity-boosting nutrient.

Mushrooms that are highest in beta-glucans include shiitake, maitake, and reishi. One hundred grams of mushrooms contains 0.2–0.5 grams of beta-glucan. Consuming more than 3 grams of beta-glucans per day shows benefits. If you have an autoimmune condition, be cautious with consuming large amounts of beta-glucan–containing foods due to their immune-stimulating properties.

SING YOUR HEART OUT

Think of the last time you sang along with your favorite song. By the end of it you felt pretty amazing, right? Your mood was elevated, your spirit felt free, and any stress you may have felt had evaporated. We instinctively know the therapeutic benefits of singing. And science backs this up.

When you sing, you engage your vocal chords, which are in close proximity to a very important nerve known as the vagus nerve. This nerve is the home of your parasympathetic nervous system (PNS). When this part of your nervous system is fully activated, your immune, digestive, and detoxification systems are operating optimally. Low PNS activation means poor immune health.

When you sing, your vocal chords vibrate and stimulate this part of the nervous system. Additionally, a study by the Royal College of Music showed that just one hour of singing in a choir boosted the release of immune cytokines (a type of white blood cell), lowered cortisol levels, and elevated levels of oxytocin in cancer patients. Cortisol is the body's main stress hormone, and it inhibits the immune system. Oxytocin is the feel-good, love/bonding hormone we all crave.

So go ahead: Put on your favorite music and sing along.

SOAK UP SOME LUNCHTIME RAYS

You may already be aware that vitamin D is very important to the function of your immune system, and that your body produces it as a result of sun exposure. But what you may not know is that sunlight doesn't trigger this response at all times throughout the day or year.

For optimal immune health, the best time to be outdoors is when the clock strikes noon. Why?

It all comes down to the relationship between your body and the sun—specifically the different wavelengths of light emitted by the sun. The most familiar wavelengths are those visible in a rainbow, which result from the light waves separating out as they travel through water droplets or a prism. Each color corresponds to a different wavelength of light.

Not all light waves reach the earth at the same time. Some penetrate the atmosphere at only specific times of day, or during specific seasons. Ultraviolet B (UVB) is the wavelength most important to your immune system. It is only when UVB waves reach the skin that the body produces vitamin D. UVB reaches the earth from early-to-mid-spring to early fall and is strongest when the sun is at its highest point in the sky (midday). UVB is virtually nonexistent when the sun is low in the sky. From mid-spring UVB levels increase, as does the duration of their availability. Levels decrease at the end of summer, and by mid-autumn they don't exist. If you live closer to the equator you'll experience higher levels of UVB for longer periods both during the day and across the year compared to the rest of the world, meaning you'll have a bit more flexibility on when you get outside for some vitamin D.

What better reason do you need to get outdoors for lunch?

EMBRACE GARLIC BREATH

Garlic belongs to a group of vegetables known as alliums that have been used to help treat a variety of conditions including fevers, gastrointestinal conditions, earaches, cholera, and even the flu. Aside from garlic, allium vegetables include onions, scallions/spring onion, leeks, shallots, and chives.

One of the main reasons for the immune effects of alliums is the compound alliin (highest in garlic). When chewed, alliin releases a sulfur compound known as organosulfur which has powerful antioxidant, antiviral, and antibacterial properties. Plants contain these high levels of sulfur in order to protect themselves against predators; it's what makes you tear up when you chop an onion and why you get smelly breath when you eat these vegetables.

Garlic has also been shown to help prevent colds and the flu in part because it helps increase white blood cell numbers when you become infected.

Aside from alliin, allium vegetables also support immune health because they contain:

- Immune-boosting vitamin C, potassium, and selenium
- Quercetin (a powerful antioxidant)
- Flavonoids, which raise glutathione levels needed for immune and detoxification processes
- Fructans (in garlic and onion only), which feed the bacteria in your gut that boost your immunity

In order to provide these benefits, allium vegetables must be chopped, crushed, or chewed so the alliin can release the powerful sulfur compounds. While there is no standard for garlic intake, studies have shown consuming 2–10 grams of garlic per day (1–2 cloves) can boost your immune system. Garlic capsules can also be taken if preferred.

If you have IBS, be cautious, as these vegetables can irritate the gut. Garlic in particular has blood-thinning properties, meaning those on drugs like warfarin should avoid it.

SWITCH UP YOUR MORNING ROUTINE

How you start your day has a huge impact on your immune health. Your body is enriched with an internal clock—your biological clock. In fact, you have not just one biological clock, but one in *every* cell. It is via these "clocks," collectively known as your circadian rhythm, that your cells know when to initiate biological processes such as the activation of genes and enzymes or the release of hormones.

This rhythm is critical to the health of your immune system and every system and cell in your body. Satchin Panda (the world's leading researcher on circadian rhythms) and his team have found that circadian rhythm disruption causes increased levels of oxidative stress (free radical damage) and inflammation, and increases your risks of developing many immune-related conditions including cancer, infections, and inflammatory and metabolic diseases. Even the World Health Organization has stated that working on a schedule that shifts frequently, versus one that stays constant, is likely carcinogenic (tending to produce cancer), and it's been shown that receiving the flu vaccine in the morning produces a greater immune antibody response than at other times.

You can build solid circadian health by timing your daily habits with what is natural for your body. How you start your day is also critical for setting your circadian clock. Here are three important habits to add to your morning routine:

- Get into natural light (outdoors, or via a bright lamp of over 10,000 lux) within the first hour of waking
- Get exercise within one hour of waking
- Eat breakfast at the same time every day

Simple habits like these can have a major impact on your immune health and risk of disease.

CULTIVATE YOUR QI

The ancient art of qigong has been shown to have powerful effects on health and the immune system. "Qi" refers to life force or vital energy, while "gong" means *work*. So, to practice qigong is to work or cultivate life force energy.

Qigong merges gentle movement, postures, meditation, and controlled breathing to strengthen, cleanse, and circulate qi. The stagnation of qi is strongly linked to the development of poor health and disease.

The main benefits of qigong associated with the immune system include:

- Healthier internal organ function
- Healthier nervous and endocrine (hormonal) system
- Immune system modulation
- Increased white blood cell count
- Pain relief
- The release of deep-seated emotions and stress

While modern science is yet to fully catch up with many of the practices and teachings of ancient traditions, there is still plenty of scientific research that demonstrates the value of qigong in supporting immune health. A core focus of much of the research has been on cancer patients undergoing treatment (e.g., chemotherapy). Results suggest that qigong can reduce stress (cortisol production), reduce fatigue, strengthen the immune system, and improve the quality of life and survival rates of cancer patients. There are different types of qigong, but the most appropriate for boosting immunity is medical (healing) qigong. Learn more about qigong and discover helpful video tutorials online.

AVOID LIGHT AT NIGHT

Your immune health and sleep are intertwined. When you don't sleep well you are more vulnerable to getting sick.

One important aspect that influences both sleep and immune health is light. The brain uses light to gauge your environment and determine the time of day. Both the type of light (wavelength) and brightness (intensity) are picked up by your brain via the eye and photoreceptors in the skin, and it then determines appropriate biological responses.

When darkness is perceived, melatonin is released by the brain. Melatonin is most known for its role in facilitating sleep but it also impacts the immune system. It modulates the immune system, meaning that it will either stimulate or suppress immune function (and can therefore have pro-inflammatory or anti-inflammatory effects) depending upon what other factors are present.

But if melatonin release is inhibited in some way your body's ability to regulate the immune system is stifled. And this is exactly what happens when you are exposed to light at night, particularly within two hours of bedtime.

Bright light and/or blue light (wavelengths) are both proven to suppress melatonin production. Blue light can come from any light source (not necessarily blue in color), but levels are particularly exaggerated from the screens of mobile devices, computers, and TVs that you may use at night.

So, for a healthy, responsive immune system, reduce your exposure to light at night, particularly blue light. This can be done through a combination of reducing exposure, using blue light filters on your electronic devices, or wearing special blue light–blocking glasses.

EAT BERRIES

Berries are a useful addition to your immune weaponry and can provide many immune-boosting benefits.

They contain immune-boosting vitamins (vitamin C), antioxidants, phytonutrients, and other immune-supporting compounds. Berries also support gut microbiota health, which plays an important role in your immune system. Aside from their general effects, berries also have unique properties. Raspberries, blackberries, blueberries, and strawberries are high in vitamin C (especially strawberries) and flavonoids. Flavonoids are powerful polyphenols found in plants that strengthen your internal antioxidant system, lower inflammation, and increase mitochondria levels. Mitochondria are cell organelles that provide the energy needed for the cells, organs, and systems of your body to function. Having more mitochondria within the cells of your body makes for a healthier and more responsive immune system. In addition, blueberries contain pterostilbene, another phytonutrient that is reported to have anti-inflammatory, cholesterol-lowering, and immune-modulating effects.

Bilberry, cranberry, and pomegranate (yes, it is a berry) have been shown to reduce inflammation and help regulate the immune system.

Pomegranates also contain vitamin E and have antibacterial and antiviral properties.

Elderberries can help cut both the recovery from and severity of colds and the flu in half! They also have antiviral, anticancer, and anti-inflammatory benefits. This explains why so many swear by the benefit of taking elderberry syrup for colds, flu, and sinus infections. Do not consume elderberries raw; they must be cooked and can be made into a jam or syrup for consumption.

Start adding berries into your diet through smoothies and yogurt or in any other way you can for a tasty way to boost your immunity.

LOOK FOR THE DEEPER CAUSE

Trying to fix your immune system either because it is underactive (e.g., you get sick frequently) or because it is overactive (e.g., you have an autoimmune or inflammatory condition) is likely to lead you down the path of superficial solutions, such as relying on the long-term use of anti-inflammatories or immune-stimulating compounds (herbs). These kinds of solutions are useful for temporary relief but fail to fully address the underlying issues behind your immune system challenges. In reality, the problem is unlikely to lie with your immune system because any presenting problem is almost always a symptom of a deeper issue.

Your immune system is always responding to its perceived environment—or it is being influenced to respond in a certain way by other factors (pharmaceuticals, herbs, toxins, health conditions, etc.). Understand that it is a system that operates within a larger network of systems. This means it is better to take a step back to consider why it is acting the way it is, rather than reach for Band-Aid solutions to specific symptoms.

By all means use supplements or foods for symptom relief as a temporary solution, but real solutions will be found by digging deeper to understand why your immune system is behaving the way it is.

QUESTION YOUR ASSUMPTIONS

You might wonder what questioning your assumptions has to do with your immune system—well, everything!

You act consistently day in, day out in accordance with your beliefs. They determine your habits and behaviors, including what you eat, how much you exercise, how much you sleep, etc. And while these assumptions about your life and the world around you may seem very real and very true to you, every belief is a result of personal experiences and/or what has been learned from others. Most of this takes place unconsciously. We all have many beliefs not grounded in hard facts.

Throughout your day you are bombarded with four hundred billion bits of information *every* second. This is obviously overwhelming, so to keep you sane, an area of your brain called the reticular activating system filters out, distorts, and deletes most of this information so that you are left with just two thousand bits. The two thousand it selects are those most aligned with your current set of beliefs. In short, your experience of life isn't something that just happens to you but something you create through your beliefs.

But what if part of what you assume is not true? And what if those assumptions aren't just false but are harmful to you? This is why regularly reflecting on and questioning what you think you know is important and relevant to your health. Some of the beliefs you have and the experiences created from them could be preventing you from making the changes needed to transform your health and immune health. For example:

- Do you deserve love, health, or happiness?
- What do you believe you need to be happy or successful?
- What do you believe about yourself and your body?

The beliefs you have in these areas and many others shape your actions, which either support or challenge your health and immunity. For example, a belief that you don't deserve happiness may lead to poor self-care and unhealthy habits. A belief that you need to earn a lot of money in order to be happy may lead you to spend all of your time working, neglecting your well-being.

Start an open and honest conversation with yourself about what you believe. Determine if these beliefs truly serve you or if it may be time to challenge them. Doing so may be the single biggest thing you can do for your immune health.

You can start to uncover some of the beliefs most affecting your immune health by using simple statements such as: "I don't _____ because _____." Now consider whether that behavior could benefit your immune health. Write down the answers that first come to you without filtering yourself.

GET YOUR DOWNWARD DOG ON

There are countless health benefits of yoga—many of which improve the health and function of your immune system. These include:

- Calming and relaxing the nervous system (stress reduction)
- Lowering chronic inflammation
- Aiding lymphatic drainage
- Toning the lungs
- Releasing toxins and mucus that build up within vital organs
- Aiding the flow of prana (life force energy)

In one review examining yoga's inflammatory and immune-modulating benefits, it was found that yoga offered many benefits in these areas, making it particularly relevant to those suffering from inflammatory or autoimmune conditions. Researchers also concluded that yoga improved function of immune cells located on the lining of the gut and respiratory tract. While there are many forms of yoga, most research to date has utilized Hatha yoga, which focuses on holding specific postures for extended periods of time.

To experience the full benefits of yoga, try practicing it as it was intended: It should be a philosophy, not just a workout. The postures (asanas) you may be familiar with are just one of the branches of yoga. In its purest form, yoga includes meditation, diet, breath (pranayama), mantras, mudras, and more. For optimal benefit, incorporate as many of these as you can. That said, the best yoga practice is the one you do on a regular basis, so find a form you most enjoy, and explore it at your own pace.

Many postures will benefit the immune system, but one of the most beneficial is Savasana (Corpse Pose). It requires the complete relaxation of the body and mind (thought). Check out more information about this pose, and how to include the practices of Hatha yoga in your daily life, online. You may also find yoga classes in your area.

TAKE A SHOT OF GINGER

Ginger contains numerous beneficial compounds with fancy names like gingerols, paradols, shogaols, and zingerone. The names of these compounds are not really important; what is important are their effects. These compounds are shown to help protect the liver, protect the body from oxidative stress (free radical damage), and provide anticancer, antimicrobial, anti-inflammatory, and anti-allergy benefits. In other words, this means that your immune system works better, you are less inflamed, and your immune system is more supported in its role to defend you from harmful microbes and cancer cells.

In one study, ginger was shown to help regulate inflammation caused by the immune system in the lungs (a common site for respiratory infection). It was also shown to reduce asthmatic symptoms, lower mucus production, and reduce overall inflammation in the lungs.

Ginger has also been studied for its benefits in supporting digestive health. Much of this research has focused on the root's ability to reduce nausea, with some research showing it to be as effective as medical drugs in doing so—minus their negative side effects.

Additionally, ginger has been shown to aid weight loss and help regulate blood sugar levels, both of which further boost immune health. The great thing about gingerroot is that it is highly versatile: You can use it in cooking, add it to tea, take it as a shot, or consume it as a supplement.

ACCEPT THE IMMUNE RESPONSE

Your body's natural response to infection can include fever (raised body temperature), inflammation (the swelling and reddening of tissue), fatigue, low mood, diarrhea, coughing, and sneezing. These symptoms are often thought of as the harm caused by the infection; however, they are not: They are the consequence of the immune system fighting an infection.

Modern medicine's solution for infections is to try to combat these symptoms through pharmaceutical drugs. And while this helps you to feel better and more capable of getting on with your day, it does nothing to support your body's efforts in fighting an infection. In fact, it means you are ignoring the body's own intelligence. These responses are the result of the immune system fighting an infection, so why restrict that? By suppressing these symptoms, you are actually putting the brakes on your own healing and recovery.

Famous philosopher Hippocrates once said, "Give me a fever and I can cure any disease." The elevation in body temperature (fever) is caused by immune messengers called pyrogens which activate part of the immune system. The fever supports the immune system to more effectively fight the virus or bacterium by creating a more inhabitable environment.

Diarrhea, for example, is the body's attempt to clear an infection from the gut, and when you suppress it you can make the infection much worse and the immune response much stronger, creating stronger ill health symptoms. And the fatigue and low mood you feel when sick are there to get you to slow down, rest, and isolate to help minimize the spread of infection. The histamine release and resulting runny nose, sneezing, or swelling are there to increase blood supply to the area and make the area more permeable so immune cells can get to the site of infection/allergen to combat the offender.

Inflammation is a response intended to promote repair and signal immune cells to come to the site of infection or injury. Acute inflammation caused by a wound or infection is perfectly healthy and should not be suppressed unless it is out of control. (Chronic inflammation is another story and needs to be resolved to avoid problems.)

You are much better off listening to your body and supporting its natural immune response by using appropriate nutrients and herbs. There are exceptions, of course, and excessive levels of any of these responses (e.g., a fever above 103°F or an allergic reaction) can in rare cases be life threatening, but in the majority, they are not.

CONNECT WITH THE EARTH

One important but less understood component of health is your connection with the earth. Both the human body and the earth are electric: They have either a predominantly positive or negative charge. And the balance of your body's electrical charge plays a crucial role in your health. When this moves away from its natural state it can create health problems. Until recent times the body's electrical balance has always been maintained through its connection with the earth, but the development of modern buildings, roads, pavements, and rubber-soled shoes has created a significant disconnection. This disconnection, along with many other aspects of modern living, has led to unnatural levels of positive charge accumulating within the body.

Because the earth's charge is negatively balanced, by connecting to it you discharge and neutralize this buildup of positive electrical charge created by modern living. This is known as "grounding" or "earthing." Studies show that grounding can:

- Regulate immune system function
- Lower stress (cortisol) levels
- Reduce free radical damage (oxidative stress)
- Improve various immune-related health conditions including autoimmune conditions, pain, inflammation, depression, fatigue, anxiety, and poor sleep

Grounding is achieved through skin contact with the earth by either walking or standing barefoot or lying on the ground. In order to work, grounding must be done on an electrically conductive surface such as soil, grass, sand, or concrete. For optimal effect, practice grounding for thirty minutes each day. You can't go wrong with simply getting outdoors and connecting with the earth.

CREATE A RELAXING BEDTIME ROUTINE

Your sleep and immune health are deeply connected. When one suffers the other is likely to do so as well. One main reason for this is because both sleep and immune health are heavily regulated by the parasympathetic nervous system. This is the branch of the nervous system responsible for rest, digestion, and recovery. If your nervous system is heavily stimulated on the opposite branch, the sympathetic nervous system (caused by stress or unhealthy lifestyle choices), your parasympathetic system will be inhibited, and your sleep and immune health compromised.

The hormone melatonin also links sleep with immunity. It is most commonly thought of as the sleep hormone since it's needed for good sleep, but it is also an important antioxidant and helps regulate immune function.

Another connection between sleep and immune health is inflammation. Inflammation is the consequence of the immune system being called into action. Inflammation has been shown to reduce your ability to sleep. This explains why those with autoimmune conditions often struggle with sleep and why illness can make it difficult to sleep. Sleep, on the other hand, helps regulate immune function (potentially reducing inflammation) and supports the repair of damaged tissue.

Doing what you can to improve your sleep will go a long way toward improving immune health. There are many habits that will help you do this, but one you can start today is to make sure you spend at least thirty minutes winding down (reading, journaling, meditating, etc.) before you go to sleep. This will slow down your nervous system, increase parasympathetic activation, and support the release of melatonin (the hormone that regulates your sleep-wake cycle).

PRACTICE GRATITUDE

It may seem almost too simple, but expressing gratitude can have count-less powerful effects on both your body *and* mind. Of its many reported benefits, those that improve immune health specifically include:

- Reduces inflammatory markers and elevations in immune antibodies
- Improves emotional health including depression, anxiety, and anger by affecting the emotional centers of the brain so that distressing emotions become less automatic
- Increases the feel-good brain chemicals serotonin, dopamine, and oxytocin
- Reduces stress in the body through the lowering of stress hormones (cortisol) and stimulation of the parasympathetic nervous system (the system that helps to slow everything down and supports the optimal function of the gut and immune system)
- Improves sleep quality and sleep duration, and reduces the time it takes to fall asleep (when practiced before bed)
- Reduces feelings of loneliness and increases feelings of sociability

There are many easy ways you can practice more gratitude each day, including:

1. **Gratitude lists.** Write a list of up to ten things you are grateful for and why.
2. **Gratitude journaling.** Write in detail about the events and experiences of your day that you are grateful for.
3. **Thank you notes/letters.** Write short notes, letters, emails, or even texts expressing your gratitude to someone.

4. **Gratitude meditation.** While meditating, focus your attention on what you are grateful for and feel the effects on your body (there are also guided gratitude meditations available online).

5. **Gratitude Kata.** Use this specific set of movements merged with statements of gratitude to help embody the feeling of gratitude, making it extra effective.

6. **A gratitude buddy.** Pick someone you can speak with every day to exchange thoughts about what you are grateful for.

Research and experiment to find which practices work best for you and your daily routine. To help optimize the effects of any gratitude practice it can also be helpful to:

- Focus on the deeper feeling that the thoughts and words provoke
- Focus on gratitude for people in your life more so than material items
- Recall the reasons behind what you are grateful for
- Come up with new things to be grateful for—or reasons you are grateful for them—during each practice
- After writing what you are grateful for, say them out loud

Above all else, be patient: The benefits of gratitude often take time. Altering your brain doesn't happen overnight!

TRACK YOUR IMMUNE HEALTH WITH HRV

When improving immune health, it can be helpful to measure immune system function. This way, you can keep track of how your immune system is operating. A simple way to do this is to measure your heart rate variability (HRV). This is a measure of the balance between your sympathetic nervous system (SNS) and parasympathetic nervous system (PNS). Low scores indicate excessive SNS activity, which means compromised immunity, as SNS activation inhibits immune function. The SNS is also stimulated during an initial immune (inflammatory) response brought about by injury, trauma, or infection. Either scenario will lower HRV and is bad news for immune health.

HRV is not a direct measure of immune health though. It has been validated in studies as a useful predictor of immune function and is used by professional athletes; however, you can improve immune health without seeing HRV score improvements.

You can measure your HRV scores easily by downloading an HRV app to your smartphone and connecting it to a heart rate monitor. Most apps will recommend compatible heart rate monitors.

HRV is also a predictor of infection risk (elevated stress) or the early stages of infection (inflammation). After recording your HRV scores for several weeks most HRV apps will provide you with a baseline score. If you see a significant drop from this score—especially for consecutive days— it will indicate either high stress or inflammation. An increase in your baseline HRV for a prolonged period would indicate a reduction in stress and improvement in immune health.

CUT DOWN ON REFINED CARBS AND SUGARS

Carbohydrates and sugar can suppress immune function. Not all carbohydrates and sugars are the enemy, but refined carbohydrates and sugars are. These are man-made, manufactured sources of carbohydrates.

Through the refinement of carbohydrate-rich foods (e.g., white flour and refined sugar), valuable fibers, vitamins, and minerals are lost. This leaves only the non-fibrous carbohydrate of the food, which, when ingested, causes spikes in blood sugar levels (hyperglycemia). When eaten for a prolonged period (over months or years) this can eventually lead to insulin resistance and diabetes.

Insulin resistance is problematic because insulin plays an important role in the proper function of immune T cells. Frequent consumption of refined carbohydrate- and sugar-rich foods will therefore inhibit healthy immune system function. In contrast, carbohydrate-rich foods found in their natural state contain fiber, vitamins, and minerals, which play important roles in slowing down the breakdown and absorption of carbohydrates/sugar into the bloodstream and increase their absorption into the cells, preventing hyperglycemia.

Additionally, hyperglycemia caused by refined carbohydrates harms the immune system because the elevation of sugar in the blood interacts with the proteins of bodily tissues (e.g., blood cells) through a process known as glycation. This interaction creates harmful compounds known as advanced glycation end products (AGEs). AGEs suppress the function of immune cells called macrophages, which play many important roles in immunity. AGEs also cause oxidative stress and inflammation (an immune response). This means the immune system is inhibited in some ways and stimulated in others, limiting the resources available to fight any potential infection.

Try to eliminate or at least cut down on the amount of refined carbohydrates and sugars you consume: Your body will thank you. You may even notice other positive side effects, such as improved complexion, fewer cravings, and more energy.

FAST TO REBUILD YOUR IMMUNE SYSTEM

Fasting has become a top health hack over recent years, in part because of the popularity of intermittent fasting as a way to lose weight or get a handle on high blood pressure. But beyond a lower number on the scale or improved blood pressure levels, many of fasting's most important benefits center around its effects on the immune system. The number one benefit of fasting is the activation of autophagy, which involves the recycling of old, damaged, and redundant cells in order to produce fresh new cells that are superior in function and health. During this process defective immune cells or their parts are replaced and toxins and pathogens are released from the cells. Autophagy can also be triggered through exercise, specific nutrients/compounds, ketosis, and even sleep. Fasting may involve eating within specific windows of time each day (e.g., time-restricted feeding, or TRF), or a prolonged period of one to five days without eating. The benefits of short-term fasting such as TRF include:

- Reduced immunosenescence (the aging of the immune system)
- Lowered white blood cell numbers (lymphocytes, including natural killer cells, and neutrophils)
- Lowered inflammation and pro-inflammatory markers
- Protection against and improvement of inflammatory-related conditions such as Alzheimer's, diabetes, atherosclerosis, and obesity
- Lowered cortisol levels at night
- Increased insulin sensitivity
- Lowered low-density lipoproteins (which transport cholesterol from the liver to the tissues of the body)
- Support for the healing of the gut lining
- Slowed progression of diabetes and obesity
- Increased weight loss
- Help in preventing metabolic and neurological diseases
- Improved effectiveness of cancer treatments

Although research is yet to clearly define the most effective time frame to practice short-term fasting such as TRF, an eating window of around 8–10 hours seems to offer the best balance between practicality and benefit. Less than six hours appears to produce mixed results, while greater than ten seems to see a significant drop in benefits.

Longer-term fasts of no food (e.g., water fasts) that last for one or more days have their own benefits for the immune system.

According to Valter Longo, one of the world's leading authorities on fasting, when we fast for 48–72 hours, we deplete liver glycogen (glucose) levels so that we rely on fat for energy. This is the state of ketosis, where the body eats up old immune cells as an energy source. As a result, immune cell levels drop but are later restored with fresh new cells once we start eating again. During fasts lasting 2–4 days the protein kinase A gene, which regulates carbohydrate and fat metabolism within the cell, is turned off, which triggers stem cells to produce new immune cells. According to Dr. Longo's research, the cumulative effect of repeated, prolonged (2–4 days) fasts is that the entire immune system can be replaced.

To gain the benefits from prolonged fasting, you must fast without food for at least three days and preferably 4–5 days for optimal effect. If you have health problems or conditions seek the advice of your doctor before fasting. Some experts recommend that longer fasts (>forty-eight hours) should only be conducted in controlled environments where different health factors can be measured.

PRACTICE TAI CHI

One great immune-boosting practice from the East is Tai Chi. Tai Chi has been shown to improve the function of many organs and systems of the body that influence immune system function as well as the immune system itself. It aids digestion and the lymphatic system (which transports certain types of immune cells and helps eliminate waste products), improves circulation and sleep, and has been shown to reduce depression.

In a study conducted by UCLA, elderly participants attended a Tai Chi class three times a week for sixteen weeks and were then injected with a vaccine for the varicella zoster virus. Compared to the control group, they showed double the immune response from the vaccine.

Another study by the National Natural Science Foundation of China looked at how Tai Chi affected the immune system of lung cancer survivors who had undergone surgery as part of their treatment. While the control group saw a significant reduction in immune cell function and an increase in stress hormones during the recovery period (the normal response to such treatments) those participating in the Tai Chi classes maintained immune function and saw no increase in stress hormone release.

Tai Chi is also proven to benefit those with immuno-compromising conditions such as asthma, fibromyalgia, HIV, rheumatoid arthritis, and more—all pointing to the effectiveness of Tai Chi in helping to regulate the immune system.

Check out more information about Tai Chi, as well as tons of easy-to-follow tutorials, online, or look for a class in your area.

WATCH YOUR COOKING TEMPERATURES

When you cook foods, particularly those rich in fat and protein, at high temperatures—or for prolonged periods—you can compromise your immune health. This is because doing so produces advanced glycation end products (AGEs). This is largely true of foods rich in animal fats and proteins and not such a problem with carbohydrate-rich or plant-based foods.

AGEs are known to cause oxidative stress and inflammation in the body, which in turn causes many of the health complications associated with diabetes (a condition of chronic hyperglycemia, which also causes AGEs) and exposes diabetics to significantly elevated risks of most degenerative diseases seen today (heart disease, cancer, etc.).

Inflammation is caused by pro-inflammatory immune cells in their attempt to protect the body from harm. These cells are called into action due to the damage to cells caused by AGEs. The immune system, now preoccupied with responding to AGEs, is less equipped to respond to any potential infection.

Studies show cooking methods that use higher temperatures, such as frying, broiling, grilling, and roasting, yield significantly more AGEs compared to boiling, poaching, stewing, and steaming. And using these lower-temperature cooking methods won't just reduce AGEs, but will also increase the nutritional content of the food eaten.

Aside from avoiding high-temperature cooking, reducing AGEs consumption can also be achieved by eating fewer solid fats, fatty meats, and highly processed foods. You can also reduce the formation of AGEs when cooking meat by marinating it in vinegar or lemon juice. Delicious *and* good for you!

LAUGH

This is one of the simplest and most enjoyable hacks for your immune system: Laugh more! There are many reasons laughter strengthens immunity. It:

- Works muscles in the face that are linked to the emotion centers in the brain and promotes the release of endorphins, which are known to stimulate immune cell activity
- Increases serotonin and dopamine levels, which help regulate the immune system
- Increases levels of T cells, natural killer cells, and antibodies, which are important immune cells that cumulatively help protect you from bacteria, viruses, and cancer
- Lowers stress, which is known to inhibit the immune system

Interestingly, even fake laughter has been shown to bring about many of the same benefits as the real thing. So do whatever you can to bring more laughter into your life: Watch comedies, read and watch humorous social media posts and videos, spend more time with your funny friends and family, bring a more playful attitude to life, or try Hasya yoga (laughing yoga).

TURN DOWN THE HEAT

A simple way to strengthen your immune system is to take a cold shower every day. This may surprise you, as, like many, you may have been told growing up (or even as an adult) that being exposed to the cold increases your risk of illness. However, there is no scientific basis for this.

Conversely there are several reasons to believe that cold exposure can improve immune system function. Multiple studies have shown that cold exposure:

- Reduces pro-inflammatory and promotes anti-inflammatory responses in the immune system—particularly beneficial for those suffering with autoimmune conditions and inflammatory conditions that compromise immunity
- Strengthens your body's internal oxidative system
- Increases white blood cell count via an increase in metabolic rate
- Increases autophagy—an important recycling process in which the body breaks down old, redundant, or defective cells and replaces them with new healthy cells (including immune cells)

Even taking a cold shower for just thirty seconds can help reduce the number of sick days taken at work. Exposing your body to the cold on a regular basis either for long periods of time at mildly cold temperatures (research suggests 59°F is effective) or for short periods at much cooler temperatures (e.g., a two-minute shower as cold as you can tolerate) can have positive effects on immune health, particularly with regard to reducing chronic inflammation. As an added bonus, research suggests that cold exposure can aid weight loss by stimulating metabolic rate.

BE ENVIRONMENTALLY CONSCIOUS

Your immune health and the health of the earth are deeply connected. In almost every situation the healthiest lifestyle choices for the planet also happen to be the healthiest choices for your immune system. Here are nine reasons why:

1. **Less toxic pollution.** Reducing your use of products and foods high in chemical toxins and heavy metals helps reduce the toxic pollution of the soils, oceans, and air of the planet, much of which also harms the plant, animal, fish, and bird populations. Many of these same environmental pollutants are toxic to your body and immune health.

2. **Less heavy metals and inflammatory meat.** Reducing your meat and fish intake improves your immune health because it helps reduce the damage caused by heavy metals (high in many fish) and reduces the inflammatory effects caused by excessive meat intake. It will also help restore a healthier balance to the earth's ecosystem.

3. **Greater nutritional content.** Going organic and/or avoiding industrially and commercially farmed plant, animal, and bee products not only significantly reduces your exposure to harmful toxins, but also enhances the nutritional content of food, which greatly strengthens your immune health. It also means you will help increase demand for such products and raise the living standards and quality of life of the animal and plant kingdoms.

4. **Reduced use of chemicals, packaging, and energy resources.** Eating a whole food diet and avoiding processed foods as much as possible helps to reduce the use of food chemicals, energy resources, and food packaging, which are toxic and wasteful to the earth, while supporting your immune health.

5. **Reduced carbon footprint.** Shopping for locally produced foods gives you a fresher, more nutritious product while reducing the carbon footprint of transporting food from far away. Outsourcing these foods internationally is especially wasteful when they can be grown in your home country.

6. **Less fossil fuels.** By moving your body more, by walking and cycling, you will use less motorized transportation which will strengthen your immune health while burning fewer fossil fuels.

7. **Greater connection to the earth.** By getting outdoors more often and connecting with nature you will receive many health and immune benefits, value the natural world more, and spend less time indoors using electricity to power TVs, computers, etc.

8. **Less light pollution.** Using less light at night is good for both you and the earth. Light pollution (especially blue light) disrupts the circadian rhythm of wildlife, including plants, birds, insects, and animals, which harms their growth and development. It also damages your health, including your immunity, sleep, and circadian health.

9. **Fewer antibiotics.** By reducing antibiotic use in humans and livestock, we can avoid the development of mutated bacteria that could potentially cause a great deal of harm to humans and animals. It also maintains a better, healthier balance of bacteria in your body.

By making better choices now, you will help secure your immune health *and* the health of the earth and plant and animal kingdoms now and in the future.

CLOSE YOUR MOUTH

Are you an "over-breather"? Over-breathing is a common but little-known consequence of today's fast-paced society that puts so many people into states of chronic stress. It takes place when you take in more air than you physically need. This may seem harmless enough but it can have big consequences to the way your metabolism—specifically the elimination of metabolic wastes—works.

The main mechanical cause of over-breathing is breathing through the mouth. The reason mouth breathing is such a big problem is because it causes you to expel too much carbon dioxide. This may sound like a good thing, as many of us were taught at school that carbon dioxide is just a metabolic waste product, but it is much more important than that. Carbon dioxide is required to move oxygen from the blood into the cells where it's needed, dilate blood vessels, open the airways, and balance blood pH levels. When you over-breathe and lower carbon dioxide levels, your blood pressure rises, cells are deprived of precious oxygen, and your blood increases in alkalinity.

Longer term over-breathing can lead to anxiety, insomnia (particularly tiredness upon waking), asthma, allergies, obesity, and fatigue. Many of these immediate and lasting effects will compromise the function of your immune system.

Therefore, making efforts to avoid over-breathing will help improve your immune health and general health in many ways. A simple way to do this is to make a conscious effort to keep your mouth closed except when eating, drinking, or talking.

INCREASE YOUR STOMACH ACID

Stomach acid produced by the parietal cells of your stomach is an important component of your immune defenses. This makes sense given that the main entry point into the body is via the gut. Any foodborne pathogens that find their way into the stomach will first need to contend with a pH of 1–2, created by stomach acid. This highly acidic environment kills the majority of pathogens. Stomach acid also aids the digestion and absorption of proteins and minerals.

Harmful microorganisms don't just arrive in the stomach via the consumption of food and beverages but also via your mouth and nose. They protect your respiratory tract from infection by coating any invaders in saliva and mucus and sending them to the stomach for extermination.

This process is negatively affected when stomach acid production is diminished (hypochlorida) or pH drops below 3. Stress harms stomach acid production, as does a poor diet (including alcohol consumption), protein deficiency, processed foods, and zinc deficiency. Some pharmaceutical drugs, antacids, a *Helicobacter pylori* infection, alkaline water, and aging also cause problems. Symptoms of hypochloridia include: acid reflux (heartburn), gas, burping, bloating, food allergies/intolerances, diarrhea, and constipation.

Many people unknowingly lack adequate stomach acid because of high stress and poor diet. If you suspect your stomach acid levels are low, address the leading causes described and also consider seeking guidance from a healthcare professional.

TRY ACUPUNCTURE OR ACUPRESSURE

The Traditional Chinese medicine (TCM) acupuncture works by releasing blocks within the body's energy pathways—also called "meridians." Each energy meridian relates to specific systems, organs, glands, joints, muscles, and other tissues in the body. There is a network of these meridians running through your body, which can be thought of as similar to your circulatory system. The meridians carry "qi" (the life force energy that creates life). According to TCM, the disruption of this qi flow leads to ill health and disease.

Acupuncturists insert special needles into the skin at key points along these energy pathways, called acupoints, to restore the energy flow through these pathways. Acupressure works in the same way except it relies on pressure instead of needles.

While modern science has yet to explain how acupuncture or acupressure works, numerous studies have demonstrated that both can benefit immunity. Research shows:

- Acupuncture and acupressure can modulate various types of inflammatory immune messengers (cytokines) and immune cells
- Acupuncture improves both conditions of excessive immune activation and immune suppression
- Acupuncture and acupressure can improve allergies and autoimmune conditions including hay fever, asthma, eczema, and rheumatoid arthritis
- Acupuncture improves inflammatory-related conditions such as irritable bowel disease and ulcerative colitis

Because acupuncture and acupressure target specific meridians that affect certain organs and glands, they have an advantage over herbs and pharmaceuticals that have a more generalized effect (and may cause unwanted side effects). A good example of effective acupressure is the Qu-Chi Hayfever Band, which is a simple band that you wear on your arm that applies pressure to the qu-chi acupoint (LI11) along the energy meridian of the large intestine, which connects to the face, head, nose, and throat. Applying pressure to this point usually reduces or eliminates hay fever symptoms. You can practice acupressure at home or on the go, or seek out a professional acupressurist or acupuncturist in your area.

TOSS THAT MOUTHWASH

You may be aware that you have an entire ecosystem of microorganisms in your gut, but did you know that such an ecosystem lives inside your mouth (your mouth microbiota)? This ecosystem features over five hundred species of bacteria and includes fungi, viruses, and protozoa. These microorganisms play important roles in maintaining the health of your gums and teeth, aiding the initial breakdown of food, and supporting your immune system against potential invaders.

The old idea that we must cure ourselves of all microorganisms has given rise to a host of habits and practices that are damaging to our health, especially our immune health. Among these is the much-celebrated mouthwash. Advertising would have you believe that this is a vital part of your oral health practices. But there is a problem: the ingredients, which can be harmful for many reasons.

Mouthwash contains ingredients such as alcohol and nitric oxide, which kill many forms of microorganisms, including beneficial ones. They also contain ingredients such as sodium lauryl sulfate (SLS), which can cause inflammation (an immune reaction) and mouth ulcers. None of this is good news for your immune system.

If you use mouthwash to fight bad breath or to protect yourself against mouth infections then the real problem isn't the microbes: It's your compromised immune system and an unhealthy balance of oral microbiota. These issues are what should be addressed. The mouthwash is a part of the problem, not the solution. But if you do insist on using a mouthwash, find one that is free from the harmful ingredients described.

RETHINK ANTIBIOTICS

While antibiotics have been instrumental in combating potentially harmful and life-threatening bacteria, they have also created major problems.

Antibiotics can kill all forms of bacteria in your body, both harmful and beneficial strains that play important roles in your immune health. For this reason, many health experts recommend taking a high-dose probiotic supplement in the weeks following a course of antibiotics. This helps, but isn't enough by itself; extra effort should also be taken to follow the lifestyle and nutritional practices that support healthy microbiota.

Another major problem of the reliance on antibiotics is that microorganisms, like all forms of life, want to live—and they will adapt in order to survive. They evolve incredibly fast, potentially into more aggressive or life-threatening strains. This is why the flu vaccine, which is developed to fight the flu strain of the previous year, can often have limited effect against the flu virus of the current year. We are always playing catchup with evolving microorganisms.

While people may benefit in the short term from antibiotics, it is creating a ticking time bomb. We are already seeing the first signs with increasing numbers of antibiotic-resistant bacteria (e.g., MRSA) in hospitals. Unfortunately, antibiotics are still prescribed at irresponsible rates. This isn't to say you should *never* use antibiotics, but it's wise to only use them when absolutely necessary. Reducing your personal use of antibiotics will support your immunity now and in the future by helping maintain the healthy balance of microbiota in your body while reducing the development of more evolved, aggressive bacteria strains.

ACTIVATE YOUR CALMING SYSTEM

Your nervous and immune systems are intimately intertwined, influencing one another in multiple ways—in both directions.

The area of your nervous system that regulates bodily processes including heartbeat, respiration, digestion, and the immune system is the autonomic nervous system. This can be broken down into two branches, the sympathetic nervous system (SNS) and parasympathetic nervous system (PNS). The SNS has a stimulatory effect on the body—the fight-or-flight response—while the PNS has a calming effect and is responsible for all things rest- and recovery-related.

Both systems can affect and be affected by the immune system. For the most part, activation of the SNS is important during the initial inflammatory (emergency) immune response, while activation of the PNS is important for immune system function at all other times. Outside of an emergency (infection or injury), you want the PNS to be active most of the time. However, due to the stressful nature of everyday life, most people spend the majority of their time in an SNS state. This inhibits PNS activity, as you can't be in both states simultaneously. As long as your body is locked into an SNS response for a prolonged period, your immune system is compromised.

Activating your PNS should therefore be the priority. The PNS is activated by the stimulation of the vagus nerve, which houses the PNS. There are many ways to do this but a really simple way to get started is to take slow, steady deep breaths in through the nose and exaggerated out breaths through the mouth or nose for a couple of minutes throughout your day.

PRACTICE THE WIM HOF METHOD

Wim Hof, also known as the "Iceman," is a Dutch extreme athlete who holds many world records involving extreme cold and breath-holding. Through the development of his methods he has gone a long way to bringing to the forefront the powerful effect that the cold and breath can have on improving human health.

The Wim Hof Method uses a combination of cold exposure, breathwork, yoga, and meditation and has been shown to reduce symptoms of diseases like rheumatoid arthritis, multiple sclerosis, Parkinson's disease, asthma, sarcoidosis, vasculitis, and several autoimmune diseases—all of which are conditions associated with immune system function.

Some of the main benefits of the Wim Hof Method connected with immune system health include:

- Stress reduction
- Improved sleep
- Stronger mitochondria
- A reduced inflammatory response of the immune system, which can be beneficial to those with chronic inflammatory conditions such as autoimmune conditions

You can learn more about the Wim Hof Method, including video courses and a free mini class, at www.wimhofmethod.com. Talk to your doctor before trying the Wim Hof Method, as it may not be safe for some.

CHECK YOUR BODY FAT

There is overwhelming evidence linking excess body fat and obesity with lowered immunity. A 2016 review concluded that obesity is linked to a decreased function of many different types of immune cells and tissues. Included within the review were discussions on how obese children have higher levels of allergies and how overweight individuals have lowered immune response to vaccines such as the flu vaccine.

One of the main explanations for this is the low-grade chronic inflammation seen in obese individuals. Fat cells have been shown to release immune proteins (chemical messengers) called cytokines. These inflammatory cytokines activate inflammatory responses within the immune system. This is problematic because while the immune system is investing its limited resources in responding to these pro-inflammatory messages, it is less capable of responding to other demands, such as when an infection arises. This provides a pathogen greater opportunity to take hold. The inflammatory response triggered by fat cells also explains why obese individuals are at a higher risk of developing degenerative conditions such as heart disease, cancer, and diabetes.

Obesity has also been shown to increase immunosenescence. Immunosenescence is the degeneration of the immune system over time. Age is the biggest player in immunosenescence, but obesity is also known to increase it. Some experts have even stated that an obese thirty-year-old has immune cells that are similar to those of a lean eighty-year-old. This explains why obese people typically get ill easier, suffer worse effects, and stay ill for longer.

Reducing body fat is one of the most powerful ways that you can improve the health of your immune system! Of course, it's important to first check your body fat level to see whether this is a good option for you. Much emphasis is placed on BMI or body weight to determine physical health, but these metrics have been shown to be unreliable in predicting cardiovascular and metabolic disease markers as they don't account for visceral (abdominal) fat levels, which are strongly linked with these conditions. Research published in 2017 showed that body fat percentage and waist-to-height ratio (WHtR) are far more accurate predictors. Healthy body fat is considered 8–19 percent for men and 21–30 percent for women, while a WHtR (your waist measurement in centimeters divided by your height in centimeters) below 0.5 is considered low risk.

You can assess your body fat levels using skinfold calipers, bioimpedance spectroscopy, or body fat scales (bioelectrical impedance analysis), although accuracy can vary. Simple things you can do to start losing body fat include eating a whole food diet, reducing intake of refined carbohydrates, exercising and moving more, reducing stress, and improving sleep and circadian rhythm health.

REDUCE INFLAMMATION

Inflammation is linked to almost every degenerative disease; wherever you see inflammation, you will find the immune system. When cells are damaged through injury, trauma, or infection, immune messengers are released. These messengers call immune cells (leukocytes) to the scene to defend the body. This is the inflammatory response.

Degenerative diseases that involve chronic inflammation include obesity, metabolic syndrome, diabetes, hypertension, hypercholesterolemia, cancer, heart disease, Alzheimer's, depression, autoimmune conditions, and more. If you suffer from any of these you are to some degree immunocompromised. When the immune system is constantly being called into action—as is the case with chronic inflammation—fewer resources are available to combat other threats, and you will likely see a weakened and/or delayed response. This provides any invading microbe or cancer cell greater opportunity to cause harm than it otherwise would. It also means the immune system will get little opportunity to rebuild, recover, and repair, which will lead to its overuse and degeneration.

Supporting the body in regulating inflammation—and, better yet, addressing the causes of inflammation—will have a powerful impact on improving your immune health and reducing your risk of disease. Inflammation has many causes, including things like chronic stress; consuming processed foods, sugar, and unhealthy fats; chemical toxins; lack of sleep; alcohol; cigarette use; and chronic exposure to electromagnetic fields (EMFs). Eating a whole food diet rich in plant foods, getting good sleep, improving emotional well-being, and reducing EMF exposure are some simple improvements you can make to help lower your levels of inflammation.

GO FOR A STROLL IN THE FOREST

Connecting with nature has many benefits to the immune system. Among these benefits, getting outside on a regular basis has been shown to lower stress, improve mental health, activate the parasympathetic nervous system (the part of the nervous system that activates the bodily functions related to recovery and regeneration), and reduce levels of obesity and diabetes, all of which are shown to have positive effects on immune health.

In Japan, the practice of Shinrin-Yoku, which translates to "forest bathing," has been shown to boost immune system function. The basics of the practice involve taking a slow, mindful walk in the forest while remaining focused on all that the forest has to offer your senses, including the smells, sights, sounds, tastes, and physical sensations.

Japanese researcher Dr. Qing Li and his team, who have studied Shinrin-Yoku, have shown that being in forest environments raises specific types of immune cells known as natural killer cells. Some of the fastest-responding immune cells in the body, natural killer cells kill cells infected with viruses and detect and kill cancer cells. Dr. Li explains in his research that the positive effects of nature on the immune system are in part due to an essential oil called phytoncide that is released by trees to help protect them from harmful microbes.

A second reason behind these positive effects are the negative ions that accumulate in such areas. Negative ions are known to boost immune system function, reduce stress, improve sleep, and kill microbes. They can be found in abundance following a lightning storm or in places such as beaches and waterfalls where you find a lot of moving water.

SPICE THINGS UP

In the Eastern world, turmeric and curcumin have been used for their health benefits for thousands of years. And with over 12,500 studies published so far, the scientific community is catching on. The active component of turmeric that produces most of its health benefits is curcuminoids (curcumin).

Curcumin regulates the immune system, including many types of immune cells. It also lowers levels of pro-inflammatory cytokines. Curcumin is a powerful antioxidant by itself, but it also stimulates the production of glutathione, the most abundant antioxidant in the body.

Better still, curcumin provides strong anti-inflammatory effects that include blocking the action of NF-kB, the protein that turns on inflammatory genes. Studies have shown that curcumin combats many immune, inflammatory, neurodegenerative, metabolic, and cardiovascular conditions and may even help prevent and treat cancer. Curcumin also supports the detoxification of heavy metals and chemical toxins, which can impair immune function.

Unfortunately, neither turmeric nor curcumin is easily absorbed in the gut, as over 90 percent is excreted. To gain from its full benefits, you will need to take curcumin in a specialized supplement form that's more effectively absorbed, such as with piperine (increases absorption by 2,000 percent) or as liposomal curcumin, curcumin nanoparticles, or curcumin phospholipid complexes. Of course, taking curcumin (or turmeric) in regular form still has benefits—they are just to a lesser degree than supplements. When taking it with food or in tea, add black pepper, which contains piperine, to help with absorption. It may also help uptake by taking it with fat, as curcumin is fat soluble.

Recommendations for dosing vary by condition, so look online to determine the best dosage for you. For general health, 500 milligrams are recommended. Consider talking with your doctor before taking it, as in some individuals it can thin the blood or cause digestive upset.

INCREASE YOUR DEEP SLEEP

Science confirms what you may already intuitively know: The better you sleep, the better your immune health will be. And while your immune system is active 24/7, research shows that the immune system is most active when you sleep—or certain components of it are, at least.

Like all cells, the immune cells need to be repaired or replaced on a consistent basis. This happens through the process of autophagy, in which old, redundant, or defective cells are recycled in order to make new healthy cells. If this process is compromised, your immune system will degenerate and function ineffectively. For the most part autophagy takes place when you sleep, mainly during deep sleep.

Improving the quality and depth of your sleep is therefore extremely important for both the optimal function and regeneration of your immune system. If your sleep is easily disturbed, you wake up multiple times in the middle of the night, or you awaken feeling unrefreshed, then you almost certainly lack deep sleep, the most rejuvenating phase of sleep. This will compromise both your immediate and long-term immune health.

Try these three easy tips to help improve your deep sleep:

1. **Turn off the lights.** Avoid artificial light sources at least one hour (preferably two) before bed. This applies to screens and bright indoor lighting in particular.
2. **Slow down prior to bed.** Avoid anything that is excessively stimulating, be it physical, mental, or emotional, during the 1–2 hours before bed. Instead focus on activities that are calming and relaxing, such as light reading, a hot bath, meditation, or journaling.
3. **Turn down the temperature.** Help keep your body cool during sleep by lowering the temperature in your bedroom to below 70°F and wearing minimal clothing.

MONITOR YOUR IMMUNE HEALTH

There are tons of ways to improve your immunity, but without a way to track your immune health, how will you know if any of it is working for you?

Luckily, you can assess and monitor your immune system at home with a few convenient, inexpensive, and non-invasive methods. The simplest way is to monitor the severity or frequency of any immune-related symptoms you may have. Symptoms may extend beyond what you would likely associate with immune health and could include the severity/frequency of:

- Illnesses such as colds and the flu
- Symptoms associated with bacterial, fungal, or parasitic infections (all kinds of infections, such as infections affecting the urinary tract, vital organs, digestive system, lungs, eyes, mouth, nose, ears, or skin; e.g., athlete's foot, toenail infections, ringworm, jock itch, etc.)
- Digestive complaints (IBS, bloating, diarrhea, constipation, etc.)
- Autoimmune conditions
- Chronic inflammation
- Migraines
- Slow wound healing
- Atopic conditions such as asthma, eczema, psoriasis, or hay fever
- Frequent/chronic fatigue
- Poor sleep quality/difficulty sleeping
- High stress levels

This is not an exhaustive list but serves as a useful guide. Improvements in any of the above symptoms or conditions you are experiencing can improve or indicate improvements in immune health.

PRACTICE LETTING GO

Stress and distressing emotions can cause not just psychological illness, but also physical illness. In this sense you can quite literally think yourself sick. While this may seem like a curse it is also a great opportunity: You have both the power to create your own stress *and* your own peace, and in doing so dramatically alter your immune health future!

One of the most powerful ways to create inner peace is through letting go, or "detaching." You form attachments every day—attachments to outcomes, people, objects, events, circumstances, experiences, behaviors, and almost anything really. When you attach to ideals, you are, by default, resistant to any alternative. Of course, this can quickly lead to problems, as life rarely goes to plan. Anything other than your ideal creates stress, usually experienced as fear, anxiety, anger, frustration, resentment, or disappointment.

The best way to release this stress and optimize your health and well-being is to let go of these attachments. This can feel difficult at first, but with practice it gets easier. Start following these steps to let go:

1. **Become aware of your attachments.** Wherever you experience stress you will find attachment. Ask yourself what attachment is currently causing you stress.
2. **Identify the underlying assumptions and/or beliefs.** Just as stress comes from attachment, so does attachment come from certain deeper assumptions or beliefs.
3. **Choose to let it go.** Letting go is an intentional act: Own your power to release something that doesn't serve you.

Try to practice these steps as regularly as possible. Eventually, letting go will feel more automatic.

CONSIDER A PROBIOTIC SUPPLEMENT

A probiotic is a live bacterium that helps keep your gut healthy, typically by improving the balance of gut microbiota. Probiotics can take the form of a fermented food or a supplement (e.g., capsule or powder). Supplementing with a probiotic can:

- Reduce inflammation and inflammatory conditions such as cardiovascular disease
- Regulate immune cell response
- Prevent respiratory (colds and flu), digestive, and gum infections
- Improve digestive conditions including irritable bowel syndrome, bloating, constipation, and diarrhea
- Improve depression and anxiety
- Improve allergies and eczema
- Improve weight loss

The benefits of probiotics to a given health condition usually depend on the strain of bacteria used. Therefore, before taking a probiotic supplement you should research online to find out which strains offer the benefits you are looking for. For general use, make sure it has a variety of strains and high numbers of bacteria (close to one hundred billion is ideal).

Despite their benefits, probiotics also have their limitations. Even a high-dose probiotic is still just a small fraction of the ten to one hundred trillion bacteria found in the body. Additionally they usually contain only a few strains, while your gut has about one thousand different strains. A large amount of the bacteria can also die between the time of manufacture and consumption. For these reasons, in order to optimize the benefits of supplementing with a probiotic, you will need to maintain a healthy diet and lifestyle supportive of a healthy microbiota balance.

MAKE DANCE A DAILY HABIT

Dancing isn't just a fun pastime: It's also great for your immune health! As seen in research into the effects of music, the immune benefits of dance seem to come down to its effects on the nervous system and in stress reduction. Regular dance has been shown to reduce stress and depression, and increase function of the parasympathetic nervous system (the part of the nervous system responsible for the rest, repair, and regeneration of the body, including the cells, organs, and systems associated with the digestive, detoxification, and immune systems). Reductions in cortisol (the stress hormone) and increases in serotonin and endorphins (feel-good hormones) have also been reported.

The more general health benefits associated with dance are also known to enhance immune health. These include:

- Improved fitness
- Creation dynamic movement (through twisting, reaching, etc.), which aids the lymphatic and circulatory systems
- Release of strong or repressed emotions (catharsis)
- Elevated mood
- Encouraged social interaction and engagement

Make it a point to get your groove on for even just ten minutes each day. Put on a favorite up-beat song and dance along at home or sign up for a regular class in a fun style that you enjoy.

LOWER YOUR ELECTROMAGNETIC EXPOSURE

There are thousands of studies showing the harmful biological effects of electromagnetic fields (EMFs). They can damage all types of cells—including immune cells. These fields come from electrical devices, which can emit three main types of EMFs: electric, magnetic, and microwave fields. The harm caused varies depending on the field's frequency (measured in hertz), its strength, and your distance from the source, duration of exposure, and health.

Magnetic fields penetrate deeper than electric fields and cause more harm, while microwave fields cause the most harm. Common EMF sources include:

- Low frequency (LF) (1–300 Hz): Kitchen appliances, TVs, computers, mobile devices when charging, hair dryers, and electrical wiring
- Intermediate frequency (IF) (300 Hz–100 KHz): TV screens, computer screens, and "dirty electricity," which results from spikes and surges in electromagnetic energy traveling along electrical wiring
- High frequency (HF) (100 KHz–300 GHz): Microwave ovens, smart meters, mobile devices, and Wi-Fi

Three to ten percent of the world population are hypersensitive to EMFs, meaning they experience clear and obvious symptoms when exposed. Of course, that doesn't mean everyone else is safe; it just means that they aren't experiencing clear symptoms—yet.

Current safety limits for EMFs are based on guidelines set during the 1970s using only thermal effects of EMFs. (Thermal effects refer to biological changes caused by elevating the temperature of human tissue.) This ignores the very harmful non-thermal effects that were known even back then. The 1972 US Navy report on 2,200 studies found 120 harmful biological effects of EMFs (many non-thermal). More recently a 2012 independent review was conducted by twenty-nine independent scientists and health experts into the biological effects of low-frequency EMFs. After examining 1,800 studies they found overwhelming evidence of their damaging effects. Hundreds of peer-reviewed studies (the gold standard of studies) also show harmful effects.

The biological effects of EMFs most relevant to immune function include: immune cell stimulation/suppression; oxidative stress; inflammation; DNA damage; damage to the membranes of cells, the gut, and the blood–brain barrier; sleep disruption; psychological damage; and gut microbiota imbalances.

While you can't eliminate EMFs completely, you *can* minimize your exposure and help protect yourself from their effects by:

- Unplugging all electrical devices when not using them—especially in the bedroom
- Keeping a 2-meter distance from electrical devices that are plugged in—again, especially in the bedroom
- Avoiding use of cordless/DECT phones
- Avoiding/minimizing microwave oven use
- Minimizing exposure to environmental stressors, including chemical toxins, pathogens, and heavy metals, which accumulate and increase your vulnerability to EMFs
- Reducing all sources of stress and inflammation
- Optimizing your natural antioxidant defense system by consuming a plant-rich diet
- Grounding to the earth (connecting barefoot with the earth) daily
- Getting out in nature often
- Optimizing your sleep
- Using proven protective EMF products

Learn more about EMFs online at www.ehtrust.org, www.electricsense .com, or www.emfscientist.org.

TAKE CARE OF YOUR LYMPHATIC SYSTEM

Your lymphatic system is an important component of your immune system. It's made up of a network of vessels (similar to your circulatory system), thymus gland, tonsils, spleen, lymph nodes, and lymph. The role of your lymphatic system is to house and transport immune cells and to help filter out waste products and pathogens. If your lymphatic system isn't working well, your immune defenses will be diminished. Reduced lymphatic health is also linked to fatigue, water retention, inflammation, and allergies.

There are many ways to improve and maintain the health of your lymphatic system, including:

- **Hydration:** The lymphatic system is 96 percent water
- **Exercise and movement:** The flow of lymph is largely created by the contraction, relaxation, and movement of muscles
- **Deep breathing:** Unlike shallow breathing, deep breathing into the diaphragm aids lymph flow
- **Massage:** Deep tissue massage helps aid lymphatic drainage, especially a specialized lymphatic massage
- **Hot and cold showers:** Alternate between hot and cold every 30–60 seconds for a few cycles, ending on cold
- **Skin brushing:** Rubbing the skin with a specialized brush helps stimulate the flow of lymph through the lymphatic system
- **Foam rolling:** Foam rolling the major muscles of the body helps to mobilize the fascia, compress muscle tissue, and break down the buildup of lymph, thereby supporting lymphatic drainage
- **Stretching:** Stretching—especially the neck, shoulders, hips, pelvis, and ankles—can help to improve the flow of lymph and release blockages and swelling

Start incorporating these practices into your daily schedule for better immune health.

COMBAT DEPRESSION

You might be surprised to learn that there is a strong link between immune health and depression—and stress is likely the common denominator. Apart from the initial inflammatory response triggered by stress, it suppresses immune function. Many people with depression also experience inflammatory-related conditions, while those suffering from autoimmune conditions (which are inflammatory) often suffer depression.

Inflammatory cytokines (immune messengers) are often elevated in those suffering from depression and affect areas of the brain associated with depression. It's not yet clear whether it's depression that triggers cytokine release or cytokine release that triggers depression. What *is* clear is that stress is proven to cause both. Additionally, insomnia, social isolation, low physical activity, and an unhealthy diet all reduce immunity and are commonly seen in individuals experiencing depression.

The causes and solutions of depression and poor immune health strongly overlap. In *Lost Connections*, Johann Hari identifies six primary causes of depression:

- Disconnection from meaningful work
- Disconnection from others
- Disconnection from meaningful values
- Disconnection from nature
- Childhood trauma
- Less influence in your own life

Each area will also weaken immunity. By building stronger connections with others and nature, doing meaningful work, living in integrity with your personal values, healing childhood trauma, and developing greater influence in your life, you are going to improve depression *and* immunity.

LISTEN TO MUSIC

It's true: There are significant health and immune benefits to listening to music! Specifically, the effect of music on the immune system seems to come via its effect on the nervous system and stress.

Studies have shown that listening to music raises oxytocin (which improves immune function) and lowers cortisol levels (high cortisol levels suppress immune function). It also improves heart rate variability (HRV) scores. HRV is a measure of the balance between the sympathetic (stress response) and parasympathetic (recovery and regeneration response) nervous systems. An increase in HRV indicates increased parasympathetic function, lowering stress. Anecdotal evidence of the benefits of music on stress and anxiety is well established with practitioners of music therapy, while some studies have even found music to be more effective than anxiety drugs at lowering anxiety. Studies also show that listening to music prior to being exposed to a stressor reduces its impact.

More direct immune improvements have also been seen in response to music, including elevations in immune cells (natural killer cells and other lymphocytes), anti-inflammatory cytokines (immune messengers), and SIgA (an immune antibody found on the lining of your respiratory and digestive tracts).

When it comes to the best type of music to listen to in order to improve your immune health, results are mixed. Relaxing music seems to have the most positive effects, although upbeat dance music has also shown positive results. A study by the HeartMath Institute comparing different types of music showed that music specifically designed to lower the body's stress response produced the best outcomes. However, what's most important is that it is music that *you* enjoy and lifts your mood.

FORGIVE OTHERS

When you hold on to bitterness, hostility, and resentment in life, you elevate stress hormones (cortisol), which suppress immune function. This is a subtle form of stress, which means you often don't notice its harmful effects. However, these emotions accumulate over time and lead to the degeneration of your body.

These unhealthy attitudes also harm your mental and emotional health and contribute to anger, anxiety, depression, fatigue, and poor sleep, which damage immune health further. Through forgiveness you can let go of these states, improving your immunity.

There is some confusion out there about what forgiveness is. Some think that by forgiving someone they are condoning their actions. This is not forgiveness. Forgiveness is the act of letting go of what you are holding on to (resentments, grudges, etc.) and encouraging feelings of compassion, empathy, and understanding. It isn't giving others permission to walk all over you. It is also not conditional on their remorse, asking for an apology, or coming from a place of moral superiority. By refusing to forgive you are punishing yourself (not the other person) with stress hormones and poor health. Forgiveness is an act of self-love and self-healing.

Aside from making forgiveness a regular practice moving forward, you can also use different tools and exercises to help you forgive events and people of your past. Useful methods include journaling, writing a forgiveness letter, or a forgiveness practice such as Ho'oponopono. Ho'oponopono is an ancient Hawaiian practice that uses a simple mantra or prayer of forgiveness and reconciliation.

Bring forgiveness into your life and notice how much better you feel. Your immune system will thank you.

GET MORE VITAMIN D

Vitamin D has a host of positive effects on the immune system, including:

- Lowering pro-inflammatory immune cytokines
- Elevating anti-inflammatory immune cytokines
- Aiding the production and activity/inactivity of almost every kind of immune cell
- Improving numerous autoimmune conditions and allergies
- Protecting against respiratory infections such as colds and the flu (when supplemented for three or more months)

Vitamin D is sourced from food or via sun exposure. Foods rich in vitamin D include fatty fish (salmon, tuna, herring, mackerel, sardines), egg yolks, liver (beef), cheese, and mushrooms (shiitake, portobello).

Plant sources provide vitamin D2, whereas animals and the sun provide vitamin D3. In order to become usable by the body, vitamin D is converted into its active form via a two-stage process: first in the liver then in the kidneys. Unfortunately, D2 doesn't convert well (D3 converts 87 percent better), making it inferior. For this reason, in order to maintain healthy levels, it is extra important for vegetarians—and vegans especially—to spend time in the sun. (This is where everyone should source most of their vitamin D anyway.)

Synthetic sources of D2 (from D2 supplements or foods enriched with D2) are the least beneficial. Dietary vitamin D should predominantly come from natural and preferably D3 sources. Studies confirm this, as naturally sourced D3 is linked with a 6 percent decrease in mortality rate whereas synthetic vitamin D (D2) is associated with a 2 percent increase in mortality rate.

So just how much vitamin D should you be getting? According to research, people under seventy need 600 IU of vitamin D per day;

those over the age of seventy need 800 IU. Some health experts recommend as much as 2,000 IU for optimal health. Consuming over 50,000 IU per day for a prolonged period is toxic, but this only arises through supplementation.

The World Health Organization also recommends that you need 5–15 minutes of sunlight directly on your face, arms, and hands 2–3 times a week to avoid vitamin D deficiency. However, obesity, dark skin, age, and sunscreen all reduce skin production of vitamin D and increase sun requirements by two or three times. In addition, if you live far from the equator (most of North America and Europe), sunlight during October to March, or outside of 11 a.m.–3 p.m., produces little vitamin D in the skin. During these times it is best to get vitamin D via a UVB narrowband light device, but you must follow the manufacturer's safety guidelines. Failing that, the next best solution is a vitamin D3 sulfate supplement. You can also assess your vitamin D levels at any time via a blood test. Blood levels of vitamin D (25[OH]D) should be 30–60 ng/mL.

BUILD A SAFE, SUPPORTIVE SOCIAL CIRCLE

Your immune system is deeply connected to your social environment through many interrelated pathways including your nervous and endocrine (hormonal) systems, your psychology and emotions, and even via microorganisms. This connection is also bidirectional, meaning your immune system is always responding to your social environment and your social behaviors are influenced by your immune status.

Because of these interrelationships it is critical to your immune health that you spend time in communities in which you feel safe and loved. Being among those who you share values, world views, and interests with can help create a feeling of security and connection. Your emotional and immune systems are used by the body to monitor and communicate feelings of safety. So safe communities play important roles in teaching these systems that you are safe. Trust and integrity within the group are also important to avoid your nervous and endocrine systems being put on red alert (suppressing immune function). Feeling valued, appreciated, and wanted by group members is also crucial.

These communities may include close family members and friends, your neighborhood, or religious, sport, interest, or study groups. The more you involve yourself within communities in which you feel safe and connected, the healthier your immune system will be. And while online groups provide lots of opportunities for connection, face-to-face interactions are extremely important to training the immune system—especially at microbial and emotional levels.

GET MORE SLEEP

Studies show that 35 percent of the US population get less than seven hours sleep each night. The numerous links between sleep and immune health tell us that if you are cutting back on sleep you are significantly compromising your immune health. It's even been shown that the effect of a vaccine in stimulating an immune response is limited by how much and how well you are sleeping before and after receiving the vaccination.

Part of the problem is that many people think that if they sleep less during the week they can "catch up" on the weekend. However, this is a myth. What plays the biggest factor in the rejuvenating effects of sleep is the amount of deep sleep (non-REM, stage 4) and REM sleep that you are getting. When you sleep longer on weekends, most of those extra minutes are spent in the lighter phases of sleep which provide little benefit to your immune system and overall health. What makes matters worse is that consistently changing sleep times has been shown to disrupt the body's biological clock (circadian rhythm), which plays important roles in your immune health.

The reality is that if you are to maintain a healthy immune system you *must* get enough sleep. The average person needs 7.5 hours of sleep each night, which usually means being in bed for around eight hours, depending on how long it takes you to fall asleep. And this sleep needs to take place at the same time each night.

SUPPORT YOUR MITOCHONDRIA

Your mitochondria play a vital role in the function of your immune system, largely because of their role in energy production. It is the job of your mitochondria to convert oxygen and food into energy that your body can use to fuel the millions of biological pathways that form every second. This fuel is called adenosine triphosphate (ATP). You have hundreds (thousands if you're in peak health) of mitochondria within every cell of your body—except blood cells, which don't contain any.

The immune system requires a great deal of energy to respond effectively to an infection. This is why fatigue is one of the first symptoms of many illnesses and infections. Autoimmune and other inflammatory conditions are examples of fatigue related to immune stimulation.

By increasing the capacity of your cells to produce ATP you can help fuel and strengthen the immune response. The simplest way to do this is by increasing the number and size of mitochondria within the cells, a process known as mitochondrial biogenesis. Mitochondrial biogenesis is sparked by many things, including regular exercise (particularly high-intensity interval training), cold exposure, saunas, fasting, cruciferous vegetables, adaptogenic herbs, and red light therapy.

Mitochondria are also highly sensitive to any changes in the environment within and in close proximity to the cell in which they reside. When they perceive danger in the form of a threat, stress, or injury, they go into survival mode, shutting down energy production in order to protect the cell from harm—a process called cell danger response (CDR). This response remains in place until the mitochondria sense that the coast is clear and normal function resumes. The CDR triggers the inflammatory response of the immune system, shuts down metabolic function, restricts energy production, and even initiates withdrawal from social contact. When CDR is triggered for a prolonged period (months or years), immunity is severely compromised and chronic (often inflammatory-related) diseases manifest.

CDR can be triggered by anything chemical, microbial, or physical in your environment, including:

- Chemical toxins and pollutants in air, water, and food
- Excessive heavy metal exposure
- Bacterial, viral, fungal, or parasitic infections
- Emotional stress
- Trauma

Minimizing these triggers is another way to support your mitochondrial and immune health.

EASE ANXIETY

No one likes feeling anxious, and anxiety has deep effects on the immune system that make it harmful to your health. These effects come largely from the stress response in the nervous and endocrine systems that is activated by anxiety. This response includes the activation of the sympathetic nervous system and the release of stress hormones, which collectively stimulate an initial inflammatory response and eventual immune suppression. Anxiety also inhibits the parasympathetic nervous system and the release of dehydroepiandrosterone (commonly referred to as DHEA) and serotonin—all of which are known to support immune system function.

Studies have also shown that there is a strong connection between anxiety and inflammation. This connection comes via the release of inflammatory cytokines, which are elevated in those with conditions such as anxiety or depression. Aside from playing important roles in immune function, cytokines are now known to affect brain function as well. This is one mechanism that explains the immune system's strong ties with your psychological well-being. It is now believed that these inflammatory cytokines play a significant role in the cause of depression—possibly the core mechanism behind it—making depression a disease of an overactive immune system (an inflammatory disease).

What is clear is that many of the same causative factors exist between anxiety is immune system disruption, therefore reducing levels of anxiety is going to have a major impact on immune system health. Simple things you can do to help reduce anxiety (and improve immunity) include practicing mindfulness, meditating, taking a magnesium supplement, taking CBD oil, getting out in nature, lowering stress, and addressing the causes of inflammation.

FEEL THE LOVE

In 2019, researchers found that falling in love boosted immune system function in women. More specifically they saw changes in a number of genes associated with the release of immune cells, particularly dendritic cells and neutrophils. It was suggested that the likely reason behind this change is a result of the body anticipating future intimate contact, which is a common route by which viruses are spread. Similar changes in antiviral genes are also seen as the body prepares itself for pregnancy.

Intimate contact with others is also known to increase the diversity and health of your microbiota (the ecology of microorganisms found on and in the body), which play important roles in your immunity and help lower stress levels, improving immune function. The biochemistry of love also releases two important hormones: oxytocin and vasopressin. Both of these chemicals play important parts in regulating the immune system. So the research certainly tells us that finding love and keeping that flame burning is good for your overall and immune health.

CULTIVATE CONFIDENCE

You can think of self-esteem as an overall sense of your self-worth—a true confidence in who you are and what you have to offer. Research tells us that self-esteem is strongly associated with your immunity:

- Low self-esteem is linked to stress and higher incidences of depression and anxiety, which are known to compromise immunity
- Low self-esteem increases the risks of respiratory infections and irritable bowel disease, which are immune related
- High self-esteem lowers markers of cardiovascular and inflammatory disease
- Drops in self-esteem lower parasympathetic nervous system function, which lowers immunity

Imagine your self-esteem as a type of emotional immune system. Just as your immune system defends you against harmful bacteria and viruses, your self-esteem fends off damaging effects of worry, doubt, regret, failure, and rejection. When unchecked these emotional and psychological "viruses" cause damage to your well-being.

In his book, *The Six Pillars of Self Esteem*, Nathaniel Branden has identified valuable principles and practices that help build confidence:

1. Be conscious
2. Practice self-acceptance
3. Practice self-responsibility
4. Practice self-assertiveness
5. Live purposefully
6. Practice personal integrity

Learn more about Branden's pillars in his book, or check out other ways to improve self-esteem online.

BREATH THROUGH YOUR NOSE

Are you more nasal or mouthy when you breathe? It might be a passive unconscious process that you pay little to no attention to, but the way you breathe plays an important role in your immune health. Breathing through your nose:

- Regulates both your blood pH and nervous system
- Traps and neutralizes particles (including viruses and bacteria) that would otherwise damage your respiratory tract and risk infection
- Produces nitric oxide, which helps reduce inflammation and aids the immune system in fighting bacteria and viruses
- Prevents "over-breathing," which causes chronic stress and many health problems including immune-related conditions

Focus on breathing in through your nose and you will do wonders for your immune health.

WORK WITH YOUR ANGER

Anger can affect your life in a host of ways—and your immune system is not exempt. Studies show that anger:

- Limits your capacity to heal
- Raises cortisol levels, which suppresses immune function
- Suppresses IgA antibodies, which play important roles in your initial response to infection
- Lowers natural killer cells (when anger is suppressed), which fight viruses and cancer cells
- Elevates inflammatory cytokines (immune messengers)
- Has strong associations with inflammatory conditions affecting digestive, respiratory, and cardiovascular systems, and joints and muscles

Anger is triggered when your boundaries have been broken. The energy of anger is there to help you reinforce, restore, or create new boundaries that aid in your happiness and well-being.

However, few actually use their anger constructively, instead lashing out or bottling it up inside. Suppressed anger is often experienced as resentment, obsessing over past events, or an inability to let go, and often results in self-medicating. It's critical to find healthy ways to work with anger. These include:

- Breathing deeply, pausing, and reflecting before reacting
- Walking away from an upsetting situation
- Releasing that energy through something creative and/or tiring, such as dance, art, or exercise
- Talking through the anger with a trusted friend, family member, or healthcare professional
- Reflecting on or reinforcing a personal boundary

Try these strategies to determine what works best for you.

CHOOSE WHOLE, REAL FOODS

Whole, real foods are foods found in their natural state—or at least as close to it as possible. They are foods that have gone through minimal or no processing. They are the foods for which your body was designed and that will support the optimal function of the immune and every other system and cell within your body. Whole foods include meat, poultry, fish, nuts, seeds, legumes, grains, fruits, and vegetables.

On the other hand, processed foods are those that have gone through a series of cooking, canning, freezing, packaging, or other preparation procedures that alter the nutritional composition of the food. Here are some of the many reasons why processed foods are harmful to immune health:

1. **Low quality.** In order to optimize profits, poor quality ingredients are used, making the food less nutritious and more harmful.

2. **Agricultural chemicals.** Since profits are the priority, the ingredients used in these foods utilize the lowest quality farming methods, which rely on high volumes of pesticides, insecticides, antibiotics, etc.

3. **Inflammatory ingredients.** Many damaged oils (e.g., vegetable oils) and proteins are used during processing, making the oil or protein highly inflammatory.

4. **Immune reactions.** Common ingredients such as soy, dairy, wheat, gluten, and eggs used in processed foods trigger immune reactions in many people (due to food intolerances/sensitivities).

5. **Lack of nutrients.** Because of low-quality ingredients and heavy processing these foods lack the nutrients needed to support good immune health.

6. **Volume of ingredients.** In order to optimize flavor, texture, color, etc., processed foods contain high amounts of ingredients.

Our bodies have evolved on meals featuring only a handful of ingredients. Eating processed foods exposes our digestive and immune systems to high amounts of natural and synthetic ingredients that can potentially create problems.

Of course, whole foods of today are much lower in nutrients than whole foods of one hundred or more years ago, simply because the intense commercial farming methods used over the years have depleted soils of nutrients and microbes and intoxicated the air, water, and soil. Nonetheless, whole foods are the most nutritionally dense foods available and the best way to source nutrients needed for immune function.

Aside from proteins, fats, carbohydrates, fibers, vitamins, and minerals, real foods, particularly plants, are rich in other nutrients we are still discovering. These include phytonutrients that regulate the way your cells and organs work to your advantage. Additionally, real foods contain microbes important for the development of your microbiota. For optimal health, aim for a diet that is 80 percent whole, real foods.

SOCIALIZE

Feeling alone and isolated is extremely damaging to the health of many bodily systems, especially the immune system. We are hardwired for connection, both biologically and psychologically speaking, and our social connections shape our immunity in positive and negative ways. Some examples of this include:

- Simply witnessing the symptoms of illness in another person has been shown to trigger an immune response
- Even the thought of getting ill has been shown to influence our decisions so that we spend less time in social settings, reducing our risk of infection
- When ill with an infection we naturally self-isolate due to fatigue, lethargy, depression, and nausea, all to protect others from our infection
- Changing our living environment, place of work, or simply the people we spend time with have all been shown to change the makeup of our microbiota, which is made up of microbes that work in conjunction with our immune system to protect us from infection
- Isolation damages mental health (increases depression, anxiety, etc.), which is known to harm immune function
- Social isolation increases inflammation levels
- Those with large social circles have been shown to be more immune to the common cold

It's clear that being social has many benefits for your immune system. What is also clear is that people have a deep need to feel safe and comfortable within those social settings. If you don't, you are likely to experience stress-related responses within your nervous, hormonal, and emotional systems, compromising your immunity. Be sure to enjoy plenty of social contact with those you like being around to boost immunity—and improve your mood in the process.

GET ENOUGH SELENIUM

Selenium is an important mineral particularly for the health of the immune system. Selenium deficiency is linked to:

- Depression and anxiety, which are known to lower immunity
- Increased risk of respiratory and viral infections, including the flu and HIV
- Significant increases in death rate in those with HIV

While the full role and mechanisms surrounding selenium's impact on the immune system are yet to be understood, what *is* known is that selenium:

- Is needed for the development, function, and protection of many different types of immune cells and immune antibodies
- Is an antioxidant
- Has anti-inflammatory effects
- Is important for lung health, and supplementation with selenium has even been found to improve asthma
- Offers protective effects against viral infections (when supplemented in high doses above minimal requirements)
- Slows down the progression of HIV
- May help improve survival rates from some forms of cancer
- Improves immune response to vaccines (when taken as a supplement)
- Is needed for circadian rhythm regulation, which plays a critical role in immune health

A minimum of 55 micrograms of selenium (60–70 micrograms for pregnant or lactating women) is recommended per day; however, for optimal immune health, you will likely need much more. Most clinical studies have used intakes of 100–200 micrograms. (Be aware that intakes above 400 micrograms are considered harmful.) Foods rich in selenium include fish, meat, eggs, lentils, cashew nuts, Brazil nuts, brown rice, sun-flower seeds, cottage cheese, mushrooms (shiitake and button), spinach, bananas, milk, and yogurt. It is always best to consume most of your selenium via food rather than through supplements.

INCREASE YOUR EZ WATER

Exclusion-zone (EZ) water, sometimes referred to as structured water or the fourth phase of water, was discovered by Gerard Pollack and his research team in the early 2000s. It is found in every cell and along the various membranes (e.g., blood vessels) in your body.

EZ water carries a negative charge, with the remaining "bulk" water of the cell holding a positive charge. The gradient between these negative and positive polarities creates an electrical or energetic potential within the cell. It is thought that this charge is then used by the cell to power biochemical processes.

The health and vitality of your body and cells are directly connected to the amount of EZ water, or negative charge, within your body, with both aging and disease linked to a low negative charge. Pollack has also suggested that EZ water may help support immune health by:

- Increasing blood and lymphatic flow (which transport oxygen, immune cells, and nutrients)
- Increasing the negative charge of the cell, which protects it from viruses and other microbes

You can increase EZ water levels in your body and cells through:

- Sunlight exposure
- Infrared and Finnish saunas
- Red light and UV light therapy
- Grounding
- Drinking plenty of water
- Eating plenty of fruits and vegetables
- Snacking on chia seeds soaked in water

WATCH YOUR IRON INTAKE

Iron is required for healthy immune function but there is a delicate balance here: Iron is needed for the production and healthy function of most types of immune cells and immune cytokines (chemical messengers), however, too much iron can increase inflammation and suppress immune function. Specifically, excess iron in the body increases levels of oxidative stress, which leads to inflammation and damage to cells and tissue, including those of the immune system. Iron is also used by bacteria and other microbes to support their growth, so an excessive intake of iron can create an unhealthy balance of harmful pathogens. We all have potentially harmful microbes in our bodies which are kept in check by our immune system and microbiota. An excessive intake of iron can suppress immunity and encourage the growth of these harmful microbes, creating health and immune problems.

Excessive iron levels most commonly arise from excessive meat consumption, iron cookware, or a genetic disposition toward iron accumulation. It is a much more common issue in men than women, simply because menstruation depletes iron levels. If you have excess iron levels, it can be beneficial to identify the causes and reduce meat and organ consumption (especially red meat and liver). Donating blood every few months will also manage levels. Iron overload is seen when intake is above 45 milligrams per day. You can measure your iron levels by requesting a blood test from your doctor or other health professional.

ASSESS YOUR NUTRITIONAL STATUS

There are tons of nutrients that are important for the optimal function of your immune system, including vitamins A, C, D, and E and minerals such as iron, zinc, and selenium. You or your diet may be deficient (or even overloaded) in one or more of these nutrients, weakening you against any potential infection.

In the same way that you need to budget and monitor your bank balance to enjoy good financial health, it is helpful to periodically check the nutritional status of your body and diet. Checking the nutritional status of your body will require the help of a trained health professional who is able to run certain tests to check and interpret your status. However, checking the nutritional balance of your diet can be done by anyone.

You can use online software such as Cronometer.com to track everything you eat and run reports to identify what nutrients may be lacking in your diet. This removes guesswork and allows you to accurately identify what foods you need to be consuming in order to ensure that you are providing your body with all of the nutrients it needs for optimal immune system function. Of course, this does not necessarily guarantee the full nutritional status of your body since there may be specific reasons beyond diet for why certain nutrients may be low (e.g., digestive issues), but it will give you a good indication as to how good your diet is so you can start making any necessary changes.

MEDITATE REGULARLY

Meditation is a simple but effective way to support immune health every day. The most obvious immune system benefits of meditation have to do with its effectiveness in lowering stress. Specifically, meditation reduces the stimulation of the sympathetic nervous system function (responsible for excitatory responses within the organs, glands, and cells of the body) and cortisol (the stress hormone) production, while increasing vagus nerve stimulation (responsible for the parasympathetic nervous system, which calms the organs, glands, and cells of the body). These changes are indicative of a body and mind under less stress.

Meditation also alters the way the brain is wired in such a way that regular meditators are more resilient than non-meditators to the stress of life's ups and downs. Meditation has been used effectively in studies to increase antibody response to vaccines, lower inflammation, increase natural killer cells, and improve depression and anxiety (both of which suppress immune function). It has also produced improvements in immune system function in studies on compromised immune systems (HIV patients, post chemotherapy, etc.), as measured by increases in T lymphocyte production. Better still, meditation protects the DNA of immune cells from damage by raising levels of the enzyme telomerase, which protects DNA from the damaging effects of stress, toxicity, and aging.

Most research into the health benefits of meditation have utilized either transcendental meditation (TM) or mindfulness meditation, however there are many other forms of meditation out there, so experiment and find what works best for you. Immune benefits may be enhanced by using a meditation that is focused on creating feelings of loving kindness, gratitude, or any other heart-centered emotion, since these internal states are known to boost immune function. The combination of these states with meditation is therefore likely to optimize your results.

REDUCE YOUR CAFFEINE INTAKE

Many of us love a cup of coffee (or two or three) to increase our energy, focus, and alertness, and even for some health benefits. However, there is such a thing as too much coffee, and from an immune perspective, consuming lots of caffeine is extremely detrimental.

Studies show that at moderate to high doses (100–400 milligrams), caffeine lowers pro-inflammatory cytokines responsible for the initial inflammatory response and also lowers immune cell levels, including monocytes, lymphocytes, and neutrophils.

Caffeine is also thought to affect the immune system via the stimulation of the sympathetic nervous system (which has an excitatory effect on the body, mobilizing energy stores, raising alertness, and preparing you for action) and cortisol (stress hormone) release, which suppresses immune function. In addition, caffeine can disrupt sleep, especially when consumed in the late afternoon or evening, and inhibits vitamin D, calcium, and iron absorption—all needed for healthy immune function.

Low doses of caffeine equate to less than 100 milligrams per day (about one half to one cup of regular coffee) while moderate doses are 300–400 milligrams (about two to three cups of regular coffee). Green tea, yerba mate, soda, and black tea contain low quantities of caffeine compared to coffee, although some black teas can contain significant amounts. Sensitivity to caffeine varies and should also be considered, as a low dose for some has a similar effect as a moderate or high dose for others.

Caffeine is sometimes used for its anti-inflammatory effects, especially by those suffering from autoimmune or other chronic inflammatory conditions. However, because it suppresses all areas of the immune system, not just the inflammatory response, the moderate to high amounts needed to lower inflammation significantly raise your risks of infection and cancer. For optimal immune health, keep your caffeine intake to under 100 milligrams per day.

HEAL CHILDHOOD TRAUMA

Unless you notice immediate effects, it may not be clear just how much past events are still affecting you. And trauma research tells us that traumatic events can affect you years or even decades later. Childhood trauma is linked to a host of illnesses or systemic damage that may take years to emerge. This is particularly true with systemic inflammatory and immune conditions (e.g., autoimmune conditions).

Trauma and other intensely stressful periods experienced during your younger years are called adverse childhood experiences (ACEs). ACEs include experiences such as:

- Physical, sexual, or emotional abuse or neglect
- Parent(s) who were incarcerated
- Alcoholic or drug-addicted parent(s)
- The loss of a parent

ACEs are associated with heart disease, cancer, suicide, alcoholism, gut disorders, insomnia, depression, anxiety, and autoimmune conditions during adulthood. One study found that for every ACE point scored on an ACE survey (with a maximum of ten points), the risk of autoimmunity increased by 20 percent in women and 10 percent in men.

Trauma also alters the brain so that pathways dedicated to learning and reasoning are weakened, while older parts of the brain associated with survival are strengthened. This weakens a person's capacity to deal with adversity. These changes are particularly damaging during childhood, when the brain is still developing.

What's more, trauma can alter genes that increase risks of developing mental health problems, obesity, drug addiction, immune dysfunction, metabolic disease, and cardiovascular disease. It can also cause other health problems, including, insomnia, addictions, and unhealthy lifestyle choices that do not support a healthy, functioning immune system.

Some forms of trauma have also been found to:

- Increase risks of colds and inflammatory conditions including asthma, cancer, and cardiovascular disease
- Elevate stress and cortisol (stress hormone) levels, not just during the event but for years later
- Increase anxiety disorders and inflammatory markers, measured years after the event

If your immune system is compromised and you suspect that ACEs may be playing a part, it is recommended that you take an integrated approach, addressing the mental, emotional, energetic, and physical components of trauma. This may include conventional therapies such as psychotherapy, counseling, cognitive behavioral therapy, and neuro-linguistic programming, as well as alternative mind-body methods such as bodywork, tantric healing (massage), Emotional Freedom Technique, Trauma (or Tension) Release Exercise, breathwork, meditation, energy healing, plant medicines, shamanic healing, Traditional Chinese medicine, and more. Check out more information on these healing methods to begin taking steps forward in your healing journey.

CHECK YOUR ZINC INTAKE

Zinc is a crucial nutrient for the immune system. It is important for:

- The healthy function of immune cells, including lymphocytes (including natural killer cells), neutrophils, and monocytes
- The poisoning of harmful pathogens via macrophage immune cells
- Regulating the initial inflammatory response of the immune system
- Neutralizing oxidative stress, which is known to impair immune function

Those suffering from autoimmune conditions often report zinc deficiencies, which isn't surprising given zinc regulates inflammation. Studies show that zinc supplementation can also reduce allergies and asthma.

Your best sources of zinc are meat, seafood, nuts, seeds (hemp, pumpkin, and sesame seeds), dairy, eggs, whole grains, legumes, and dark chocolate. Vegetarians and vegans typically have much lower levels of zinc than those who eat meat and/or animal byproducts, because many plant sources of zinc are less easily absorbed due to their levels of phytate, which blocks the absorption of minerals including zinc. You can break down phytates by sprouting or soaking plant sources (e.g., grains, legumes, nuts, and seeds) for about twenty-four hours before consuming them and by cooking them (e.g., grains and legumes). Although it is recommended that you get zinc primarily from your diet, supplements are also available.

Daily recommendations for zinc are 11 milligrams for men and 8 milligrams for women (11–13 milligrams for women who are pregnant). While zinc toxicity is rare, avoid consuming 50 or more milligrams per day, as excessive intake disrupts the absorption and function of iron, another important mineral.

TRUST YOUR PSYCHOLOGICAL IMMUNE SYSTEM

There is a strong connection between your immune state and psychological state. Studies show that stress and anxiety have powerful immuno-suppressive effects.

Luckily, each of us is armed with mechanisms built into our psyche that support us in handling stressful situations. One such mechanism is called the psychological immune system (PIS). The PIS is a series of psychological strategies we unconsciously use to navigate stressful events. The most relevant strategy to immune health relates to how you might expect to respond emotionally to future situations. Social psychologists have found that people are notoriously bad at predicting their emotional response to both minor and major life events.

It's normal to expect that the most difficult events (job loss, relationship breakups, etc.) would provoke the most intense and difficult emotions that take the longest time to pass. However, that is not what the psychologists found. What they discovered is that when emotional stress reaches a certain threshold, the PIS kicks in to protect you from becoming emotionally overwhelmed. This built-in system of resilience enables you to handle difficult circumstances better than you might expect.

Instead of stressing and building anxiety over anticipated events, remember that you have this natural ability, your PIS, that enables you to be stronger and more resilient than you may give yourself credit for. Keeping this in mind will strengthen your immunity by helping you let go of anxiety associated with events that may or may not happen in the future.

TRY OUT DIFFERENT TYPES OF FASTING

Fasting, or intentionally abstaining from calories for a certain period of time, offers a number of benefits to the immune system, including:

- Autophagy (the recycling of cells and cell parts)
- Reductions in inflammation and inflammatory markers, including pro-inflammatory cytokines, c-reactive protein, and low-density lipoprotein
- Reducing oxidative stress
- Weight loss (which lowers chronic inflammation)
- Improving insulin sensitivity and blood sugar regulation
- Aiding gut health (gut lining is repaired)
- Helping prevent cancer
- Possibly improving autoimmune and neurodegenerative diseases

There are many types of fasting out there, with some producing better results than others. Longer fasts likely provide greater benefits, but shorter fasts are more practical and can be done more often. Popular types of fasting include:

1. **Time-restricted feeding (TRF).** TRF involves fasting for 12–16 hours every day.
2. **Intermittent fasting (IF).** IF involves alternating between set cycles of fasting and eating. There are several methods of IF, including 5:2 (five days eating a normal diet and two days eating 700 kilocalories), alternate-day fasting (eating 500 kilocalories every other day and eating a normal diet on the off days), TRF, and 16:8 (TRF done with sixteen-hour fasts).
3. **Water fasting.** This fast lasts for 24–72 hours (or in some cases much longer) and can be done on a regular basis. Fasts for three or more days provide the most benefits—especially to

the immune system—but fasts of 24–48 hours still offer many benefits.

4. **Fasting Mimicking Diet (FMD).** Developed by fasting researcher Valter Longo, this diet mimics the health benefits of a 4–5 day water fast without the challenge of not eating for five consecutive days. It involves following a low-calorie, low-protein, vegan diet for five days. The official version of the diet is completed using FMD meal kits made to specific macronutrient ratios and calories. It's possible to follow the dietary guidelines by making your own meals with a little bit of nutrition knowledge or unofficial meal plans found online.

Try out the different types of fasting to determine which may be best for your needs and lifestyle. Be sure to end a fast gently, especially if doing a longer fast. This is done by focusing the first few meals or days on eating light and consuming only broths, juices, fruits, and vegetables and avoiding heavily processed foods.

SWITCH TO UNPROCESSED WHOLE GRAINS

Grains can be a nutritious source of immune-boosting nutrients, including:

- Minerals (particularly zinc, iron, and magnesium)
- B vitamins
- Phytonutrients (including sterols and polyphenols)
- Fiber
- Antioxidants

Not all grains have a positive effect on immune health, however. Refined grains—for example, white flour and white rice—are grains that have typically had their germ and bran removed, leaving just their endosperm (the starch). Refining grains removes about 25 percent of the protein and up to 70 percent of their beneficial nutrients (fiber, vitamins, minerals, and phytonutrients). Not only are these grains depleted of nutrients, but they also break down in the gut extremely quickly, causing spikes in blood sugar. When processed grains are consumed on a frequent basis, these sugar spikes can lead to insulin resistance and diabetes, which impair immune health. Grains can also be processed in other ways, beyond refining, to alter their form (e.g., breakfast cereals). This process uses extreme heat and pressure, which damages the proteins, fats, and/or fibers, making them inflammatory.

Unprocessed whole grains are grains that have neither been refined nor processed. This ensures nutrient content is maintained, including phytonutrients such as polyphenols, which upregulate anti-inflammatory and antioxidant pathways, improving immune health. Polyphenols alongside fiber and resistant starch found in these grains also support the development of a healthy gut microbiota, which has important roles in supporting your immune system.

When consuming any form of grain, it is useful to cook it well to help break down the phytates that can block the absorption of minerals.

PRAY

It may sound unusual, but daily prayer can help improve your immune system!

Of the more immediate effects, prayer appears to affect the body and mind in similar ways to meditation, mindfulness, yoga, Tai Chi, and qigong. It lowers the effects of stress, including slowing down the nervous system and heart rate, and lowers cortisol levels (the stress hormone), effects that are associated with better immune health.

Observational studies show that frequent prayer benefits those suffering from mental health conditions including stress, depression, and anxiety. Prayer improves psychological well-being by adding meaning to one's life and reduces the stressful impact of life's difficulties. Those who pray regularly have been shown to have fewer depressive symptoms, higher self-esteem, and less severe asthma.

Prayer also helps you develop self-control. A series of studies found that those who prayed regularly were much less likely to drink heavily and one study even showed that four weeks of prayer reduced alcohol intake by 50 percent. This suggests that developing self-control (be it through prayer or other means) has positive effects on lifestyle choices that affect immune health.

While there are many ways to pray, studies show that prayer focused on gratitude or concern for others is more effective in improving states of depression. This makes sense, as studies outside of prayer demonstrate that adopting states of kindness, compassion, and gratitude enhance mental and immune health. Consider making prayer a part of your routine.

PRACTICE MINDFULNESS

Mindfulness is the act of bringing awareness to the present moment—to your thoughts, emotions, body sensations, and environment in the here and now. Through mindfulness, you allow yourself to experience anything that enters your awareness, without judgment or assessment. The practice of mindfulness is a simple but effective way to lower stress and build immunity at any moment of the day.

Immune benefits of mindfulness include:

- A reduction in stress response, as seen through lowered cortisol levels and an increased activation of the parasympathetic nervous system, which is responsible for your non-inflammatory immune response
- A reduction in the inflammatory immune response
- Increased healing from wounds
- Increased levels of telomerase (an enzyme that helps protect the telomeres that are found at the end of your strands of DNA) in immune cell DNA; increases in telomerase mean that the DNA of your immune system is better protected from wear and tear
- Lower levels of anxiety and depression
- Increased stress resilience

Research into the effect of mindfulness on the immune system has mainly used meditation, which is just one way to practice mindfulness. Mindfulness can be practiced at any opportunity during specific moments, or everyday activities like exercising, washing dishes, cooking, eating, or showering. During these activities, you'll want to pay close attention to everything you see, taste, touch, smell, and feel inside and out (your thoughts, body sensations, and emotions). Avoid getting caught up in thinking, judging, labeling, defining, or assessing anything. Know that every time you practice mindfulness you are lowering stress and giving your immune system a much-needed boost!

PLAY A MUSICAL INSTRUMENT

Like with many studies into the effects of listening to music on the immune system, playing a musical instrument has been shown to lower cortisol, stress, anxiety, and depression—all of which diminish your immunity.

One of the most researched instruments in respect to immune function is the drum. One study found that drumming increased natural killer cell activity, lowered cortisol levels, and increased lymphokine-activated killer cell activity, all mechanisms used by the body to combat cancer and illness. Another study found that drumming reduced the inflammatory immune response both immediately following playing and for several weeks afterward.

Other studies have found that playing music increases levels of IgA, an important antibody found on the mucosal lining of the gut and respiratory systems, as well as natural killer cells, important immune cells that help keep invading pathogens and cancer cells in check.

What better excuse to dust off your guitar, or finally learn to play the piano?

GET MORE MAGNESIUM

Magnesium is one of the most important nutrients for your health and is involved in over three hundred metabolic functions, including many involving the immune system:

- Low levels of magnesium elevate pro-inflammatory cytokines (immune messengers)
- Magnesium helps regulate levels of various immune cells
- Magnesium supports healthy immune organs including the thymus and spleen

The importance of magnesium is also demonstrated via its effects on immune-related conditions:

- Magnesium deficiency elevates oxidative stress and inflammation while reducing mitochondrial function, all of which will impair immune function
- Magnesium deficiency is linked to several conditions known to damage or reflect poor immune function, including insulin resistance, asthma, cancer, depression, and anxiety
- Magnesium supplementation can improve chronic inflammation, insulin resistance, metabolic syndrome, skin allergies, insomnia, depression, and anxiety

Magnesium deficiency is one of the most common deficiencies, affecting about 50 percent of Western society. The most common causes of deficiency include emotional stress, poor absorption (digestive issues), aging, chronic disease, kidney problems, or simply a lack of magnesium in the diet.

The recommended daily intake of magnesium is 420 milligrams for men and 360 milligrams for women. Magnesium-rich foods include pumpkin seeds, dark chocolate, black beans, quinoa, almonds, cashews, avocado, leafy greens (spinach, swiss chard), red meat, and seafood (salmon, mackerel).

You can boost magnesium levels by increasing your intake of magnesium-rich foods (preferable) or by taking a magnesium supplement. The most easily absorbed forms of magnesium are organic (e.g., aspartate, citrate, fumarate, malate, acetate, ascorbate, taurate, or gluconate).

HUG YOUR LOVED ONES

A simple, enjoyable way you can boost your immune system is through hugging family and friends. It's true! Hugging provides many health benefits and boosts immunity:

- One study found that hugging lowered risks of infection and symptoms were less severe among those who got sick
- Hugs stimulate the release of oxytocin, serotonin, and dopamine, which elevate mood and regulate immune function
- Hugs apply gentle pressure on the breastbone, stimulating the thymus gland, which stores and releases many of your lymphocyte immunes cells
- Hugs lower levels of cortisol (the stress hormone), stress, and anxiety—all immunosuppressants
- Hugs deactivate the area of the brain that responds to threats and notifies your nervous system that you are safe, allowing you to relax and the immune system to function better
- Hugs encourage skin-on-skin contact, during which you exchange immune antibodies and skin microbiota with the other person, which helps develop and regulate your immune system
- Hugs lower depression and improve sleep

One important point to keep in mind is that hugs must be with someone you trust in order to experience these benefits. While there is no exact number of hugs determined for optimal immune health, the general consensus is that more is better. Famous family therapist Virginia Satir is often quoted as saying, "We need four hugs a day for survival. We need eight hugs a day for maintenance. We need twelve hugs a day for growth."

FORGET ABOUT MODERATION

It is often believed that consuming foods and beverages that are harmful to human health is part of a healthy lifestyle plan just as long as it's in moderation. This viewpoint is flawed.

Firstly, the term "moderation" is highly subjective: What may be moderate for you may be excessive for someone else. Secondly, studies show that when recalling our choices we made that day or previous days, we can be highly inaccurate. We may then use this inaccurate data to justify our future choices, leading to excessive unhealthy habits that we think are moderate.

Thirdly, and most importantly, "everything in moderation" is a false economy. There are many harmful or potentially harmful foods and beverages you may be consuming in "moderation," such as alcohol, caffeine, refined sugar/carbohydrates, inflammatory fats, meat (in excess), processed foods, common food allergens (soy, dairy, wheat, gluten, etc.), and more. If you consume many of these foods in moderation, that makes for an excess of harmful foods. Every one of these foods and drinks triggers inflammation and impairs immunity. If you then include other common lifestyle choices known to harm immunity, such as stress, smoking, sedentary living, late nights, chemical toxin exposure, and electromagnetic stress, it's easy to understand why everything in moderation is a dangerous idea.

Ditch this term once and for all and focus on reducing the amount of harmful (or potentially harmful) foods you consume, as well as other harmful lifestyle habits.

EMBRACE THE SEASONS

Did you know your immune system works seasonally? It's true! The types of microbes and threats to our health vary by season. For example, the winter and autumn see a rise in viruses. This is likely because there is much less sunlight, which means that there is much less UV light to kill viruses, and low to no UVB light, which is needed for vitamin D production in the skin. The risk of catching a virus is therefore much greater in the colder months, but is that necessarily a bad thing?

Some experts suggest not. There is a school of thought that some infections actually help develop the immune system, which benefits us later in life. For example, catching the virus that causes chicken pox develops our immunity to both chicken pox and shingles (which is caused by the same virus). Shingles, which develops later in life, can cause blindness and is far more deadly, while getting chicken pox as a child is rarely dangerous. Some experts also believe that certain mild childhood infectious "diseases" are protective against infectious and/or degenerative diseases later in life.

Of course, this doesn't mean that winter needs to be a time of frequent illness. A healthy, fully responsive immune system means you can acquire viruses without experiencing illness. After all, the symptoms of infection are the result of the immune response, not the microbe. If the immune system is healthy and functional, you may acquire a virus with only minor or even no symptoms. This means you get all the benefit of long-term immunity and protection against serious infections and diseases without getting "sick."

Seasonality is also reflected in food. Plants naturally develop the nutrients and compounds inside their fruit and/or roots that they need to fend off pathogenic microbes found in their geographical and seasonal environment. This is also true of their fibers. Different fibers support different strains of symbiotic bacteria that provide nutrients and protection to the plant against pathogenic microbes. These fibers support your gut microbiota in the same way. This essentially creates seasonality within your gut microbiota and immune system so that you are better prepared for any pathogenic microbes. For instance, fruit fibers support different bacterial strains compared to leafy greens or mushrooms. When you eat out-of-season, non-local, heavily processed foods you rob yourself of this natural protection.

Embrace the seasons in every way you can and you will develop a healthy, well-balanced immune system. Start by eating local, seasonal produce from local farmers and providers.

EXERCISE DAILY

Exercise is critical to your health, there is no argument on that. And it can have positive effects on your immune health too:

- Exercise helps regulate every kind of immune cell
- Muscle contractions during exercise release high amounts of muscle-specific immune messengers called myokines that regulate inflammation
- Exercise lowers systemic inflammation common to cardiovascular and metabolic disease and has a generalized anti-inflammatory effect for all
- Exercise increases telomere length in immune cell DNA, which helps protect it from the effects of stress and aging
- Exercise improves the health and diversity of gut microbiota, which helps regulate inflammation and the immune system and defend the body from harmful pathogens
- Exercise improves antibody response to vaccines
- Exercise slows down the aging of the immune system (known as immunosenescence)
- Exercise produces acute low levels of free radicals that strengthen your internal antioxidant system
- Exercise is protective against many of the most common inflammatory and immune-related conditions seen today, including cancer, diabetes, obesity, metabolic syndrome, and atherosclerosis
- Exercise aids weight loss and improves most diseases of chronic inflammation (e.g., autoimmune conditions)
- Exercise strengthens the vagus nerve, which regulates immune response

- Studies have found that regular physical activity can cut the duration of time spent ill with colds and flu by almost half, while infection rates are also significantly reduced

One hundred fifty minutes of moderate exercise or seventy-five minutes of high-intensity exercise each week is recommended. Try to exercise every day. If you are just starting out, you can also start by exercising every other day for short periods.

SMILE MORE

Don't be fooled by its simplicity: Smiling has many benefits!

Firstly, its direct effect on the immune system includes raising levels of immune antibodies and immune cells. This is because a smile is one of the first signs of humor, so when your brain senses your smile it mounts the same immune response as it does to humor. Secondly, smiling activates nerves in the face that turn on areas of the brain that elevate your mood and stimulate the release of serotonin and dopamine—feel-good hormones that regulate the immune system. Finally, smiling is proven to mitigate the effects of stress: the antithesis of immune health.

And smiling isn't just good for your personal immune health. It's also good for those around you. Mirror neurons found within your brain allow you to imitate the behavior of those around you, including their emotional state. So when you see someone else smile these neurons allow you to gain from the same emotional and biochemical effects. We all know how contagious a smile can be. By smiling more, you will elevate the mood and immune health of those around you as well as yourself!

A really simple but powerful way to bring the benefits of smiling into your life is to begin your day with a smile as soon as you wake up. It will set the tone for the day and give your immune system a vital boost. Hold the smile for just long enough for your brain and body to get the message—thirty seconds should be sufficient. Like anything else it becomes easier and more effective with practice.

CRUNCH ON CRUCIFEROUS VEGETABLES

Of all food groups, especially within the vegetable family, some of the best foods you can eat for health and immune benefits are cruciferous vegetables. Why? They are packed full of immune-boosting nutrients and compounds known to enhance immunity, including:

1. **Vitamins.** Cruciferous vegetables are high in vitamins C and E, important to immune function.
2. **Fiber.** Cruciferous vegetables are high in fiber, which feeds your gut microbiota.
3. **Chlorophyll.** Chlorophyll contained in these vegetables has wound, immune, and anticancer benefits.

Cruciferous vegetables are rich in phytonutrients such as polyphenols and glucosinolates (compounds that contain sulfur), which provide antimicrobial, anticancer, anti-inflammatory, antioxidant, and detoxification benefits and help to protect cell DNA, including that of the immune system.

Glucosinolates also activate the immune system in the gut. These compounds are broken down in the gut to indole-3-carbinol (I3C) and eventually diindolylmethane (DIM). DIM activates cells within your gut lining which turn on specialized lymphocyte immune cells within the gut. It is believed that this mechanism is there because when you eat, you are most vulnerable to infection—especially because unlike anywhere else within the body, your gut lining is just one cell thick. By activating the immune system through food, the body has developed a smart way to protect itself when most vulnerable without wasting energy when it isn't needed.

Cruciferous vegetables include beet greens, bok choy, broccoli, Brussels sprouts, cabbage, cauliflower, collards, horseradish, kale, mustard greens, radishes, red cabbage, turnip greens, and watercress. Aim to consume 2 cups of cruciferous vegetables every day.

CURB A SMOKING HABIT

It's no surprise that smoking is incredibly bad for both your immune and general health:

- Smoking increases pro-inflammatory cytokines and has other inflammatory effects
- Smoking disrupts the function of all types of immune cells
- Cigarettes contain several heavy metals including nickel, cadmium, arsenic, and lead, all of which can accumulate within the body and damage immune cell function
- Cigarettes contain several thousand different chemicals, some of which can harm many areas of your health including your immune health
- Nicotine found in cigarettes stimulates the sympathetic nervous system (which activates the stress responses in the body, elevating heart rate, blood pressure, respiratory rate, and more) while suppressing immune system function
- Frequent exposure to cigarette smoke can cause infections, numerous types of cancer, and respiratory and cardiovascular diseases
- There is strong evidence that smoking worsens already-established immune-related conditions including diseases of chronic inflammation and autoimmunity (rheumatoid arthritis, lupus, COPD, and psoriasis)

Given the harm caused by cigarettes many have resorted to vaping, but is this any better? Evidence suggests that while it is better for you than smoking cigarettes, it is still very harmful. From the perspective of the immune system:

- Vaping limits the response of immune cells to infection in both intensity and breadth
- It still contains nicotine with all of its harmful immune health effects
- It increases inflammation within the lungs
- It contains chemicals that very little is known about
- The electromagnetic stress emitted by e-cigarettes is potentially harmful

The bottom line is that stopping or at least cutting down on smoking cigarettes and/or vaping is one of the most beneficial things you can do for your immune system.

BE CAUTIOUS OF 5G

Introduced for its technological benefits (e.g., the Internet of Things, mass surveillance, etc.), 5G is the fifth generation technology standard for cellular networks, implementing service areas across the world that connect to any mobile device. One of the main differences between 4G and 5G is greater speed—up to ten gigabits per second.

On the surface this may sound great; however, the harmful effects of electromagnetic fields (EMFs), particularly on immune health, are well researched, and 5G takes these effects to the next level. 5G technology uses mainly higher frequencies than earlier technology (1G–4G uses 600 MHz–6GHz, while 5G uses 6 GHz–300 GHz). It will also use 600 MHz–6 GHz, but at higher intensity levels due to increasing demands for data. The higher frequencies above 30 GHz are called "millimeter waves" and are up to one hundred times stronger than 4G waves. These millimeter waves require a lot more cell towers positioned at more frequent points in our environment than previous cell towers, as they struggle to penetrate trees, buildings, or even rain.

This has important ramifications because the severity of EMF effects is in direct proportion to your distance from a tower. The closer you are, the stronger the signal and the more harm it can cause. Many studies demonstrate that both continuous and pulsed millimeter waves harm bodily tissues. In fact, millimeter wave technology at the frequencies used by 5G (95 GHz) are used by the US military at higher power outputs to disperse crowds. They work by causing burning sensations on the skin. As yet there is not enough research done to specify the exact immune effects of 5G; however, research into the biological effects of other forms of EMFs and millimeter waves provides reasons to be cautious.

Low-intensity millimeter waves have been used in medical procedures in Russia for decades to treat cardiovascular and metabolic conditions.

While these procedures produced beneficial outcomes, they were not pulsed and were only used for a short duration. This therefore doesn't rule out the harmful effects of long-term exposure.

Protect your immune system and your health from the harmful effects of 5G by taking good care of your health, minimizing your exposure to all forms of stress (emotional, chemical, etc.), eating a phytonutrient-rich diet, taking an N-acetyl cysteine supplement, practicing grounding, minimizing your exposure to all forms of EMFs as much as possible, and taking no part in the Internet of Things (the connection of all devices that can speak to one another). Avoid these devices as much as you can. You can learn more about 5G and its effects at www.5gappeal.eu.

TAKE ECHINACEA FOR VIRAL INFECTIONS

Echinacea is an herb commonly taken to help combat colds. Research has revealed that it:

- Increases activation of immune cells including macrophages and dendritic cells, which are involved in the initial response of the immune system to infection
- Has antioxidant and anti-inflammatory effects, especially within the respiratory tract
- Is mainly used to combat viruses affecting the upper respiratory tract (particularly the common cold), although it has been reported to have benefits against some strains of yeast, bacteria, and parasites

Evidence of echinacea's effectiveness at combating infections is mixed. Some studies show that it is useful in preventing infection while others show that it is more useful in reducing severity of symptoms or duration of illness. Still others show its benefits are in fighting infections, especially during the early stages. In general, most research seems to point to its benefit in the early stages of infection. Because of some of its mechanisms of action there may be complications with long-term use.

The effectiveness of echinacea supplements varies because of differences between extracts and the part of the plant used. Extracts may include the whole plant or just parts of the plant, such as the roots, flowers, leaves, or stems. These can be taken via tinctures, teas, sprays, capsules, tablets, juices, dried roots, or dried leaves. Additionally, there are three species of echinacea plant used in supplements. Because of all these variables and differences in effectiveness it is best to experiment in order to find which works best for you.

Those with autoimmune conditions or those taking immunosuppressants should not take echinacea.

CONSIDER COLOSTRUM

Colostrum is the first milk fed to a baby mammal following birth. Its main purpose is to give the baby an immune boost. It is rich in immune antibodies (IgA, IgG, and IgM), vitamins, minerals, fats, carbohydrates, disease-fighting proteins (e.g., lactoferrin), and digestive enzymes. It is commonly used as a nutritional supplement, sourced from the first milk of a mother cow.

Colostrum boosts immune cells (e.g., monocytes and T cells) within one hour of taking it and is particularly effective at preventing respiratory infections, such as colds and flu. One study even found that it was three times more effective than the flu vaccine at reducing the number of days of flu infection.

Due to its high content of antimicrobial lactoferrin, colostrum may also be effective at reducing diarrhea. Its lactoferrin content might also explain its effectiveness in reducing intestinal permeability (leaky gut).

Colostrum is particularly useful for athletes and very active individuals prone to colds and flu, which are often caused by high volumes of exercise known to suppress immune function, particularly along the mucosal lining of the respiratory and digestive tracts. Studies using colostrum in these groups found that it:

- Significantly elevated SIgA levels (the main antibody found along the mucosal lining)
- Reduced respiratory infection rates
- Reduced exercise-induced immune depression

Depending on the source, colostrum supplements may contain pesticides, antibiotics, and other synthetic chemicals. For this reason, only use high-quality colostrum from reputable sources. Do not use colostrum if you are allergic to dairy.

PRACTICE SELF-LOVE

One of the most effective, and likely surprising, ways to improve your immune function is by loving yourself. There are many ways this works:

1. **Self-compassion:** Being kind to yourself increases self-love and reduces depression, boosting immune health
2. **Self-care:** Simple practices of care, including regular exercise, eating a healthy diet, and getting plenty of sleep, build a sense of high regard for your well-being and improve immune health
3. **Addiction:** Unhealthy addictive behaviors, including drug and alcohol abuse and overeating, often arise when self-love is lacking, and they weaken immunity
4. **Self-criticism:** Harsh words and attitudes toward oneself arise when self-love is lacking and can lead to overworking and a lack of self-care, which harms well-being and immune function
5. **Mental health:** Anxiety and depression are both known to suppress immune function, and a lack of self-love often contributes to their development

One study compared the effects of exercises designed to increase self-compassion and self-love to exercises that were either emotionally neutral or produced self-criticism. Researchers found that the participants who practiced the self-love exercises had significantly lower heart rates and higher levels of heart rate variability (HRV). Higher HRV indicates greater activation of the parasympathetic nervous system (responsible for the recovery and regeneration of the body, including systems such as the digestive, immune, and detoxification systems), and lower heart rates indicate lower levels of stress, both of which improve immune system function.

So how do you build a stronger sense of self-love? Here are a few simple ways to start:

1. **Self-care:** Get into the habit of doing caring things for yourself each day, including looking after your hygiene, eating well, drinking water, and enjoying a favorite activity.
2. **Self-compassion:** Let go of harsh self-judgment or criticism, accept your imperfections, and speak to yourself in the kind and positive ways you would speak to a close friend or family member.

You can also begin improving your sense of self-love by visiting a mental health professional. Investing in your mental health is investing in your immune health.

LIVE WITH PURPOSE IN SERVICE TO OTHERS

Did you know that there are two types of happiness? They are eudaemonic and hedonic. Eudaemonic happiness is achieved through good character or spirit and involves pain and adversity. Hedonic happiness is achieved through self-pleasure or self-indulgence and involves avoiding pain and adversity. Hedonic happiness is short-lived and is focused on having a good time. Eudaemonic happiness is longer term and arises out of the meaning, purpose, and service that come from striving to be the best version of yourself.

Hedonic happiness is what we are sold every day via advertising, movies, and TV shows promising money, sex, beauty, and more. Eudaemonic happiness emphasizes the pursuit of happiness through health, safety, friendships, culture, music, art, and service to others.

Of the two, only eudaemonic happiness positively affects immune health. In studies, happiness type has been assessed alongside genes linked to inflammatory and antiviral activity. Eudaemonic happiness is shown to lower inflammatory gene activity and raise antiviral gene activity. The opposite pattern occurs with hedonic happiness—the same response you'd expect from chronic stress. Another study used the same metrics via a nine-month intergenerational program, during which participants assisted young school children with learning difficulties. At the end of the program increases in eudaemonic happiness were linked to elevations in antiviral gene activity and drops in inflammatory gene activity.

It's clear that living a life focused on seeking happiness through meaningful pursuits that allow you to grow and serve others strengthens the health of your immune system, while focusing life on self-indulgence damages it.

PACE YOURSELF

Although it is a rare problem for most people, too much exercise harms your immune system. Exercise strengthens your immune system but too much suppresses the function and production of many types of immune cells:

- Exercising at moderate-high intensity for greater than ninety minutes harms the mucosal lining of the gut, which keeps harmful invaders out of the body, and suppresses immune function for up to three days
- SIgA (the main immune antibody on the mucosal lining) is temporarily reduced by high volumes of exercise (e.g., training for and running a marathon)
- Over-exercise damages gut microbiota balance
- Endurance exercise elevates cortisol (the stress hormone), which is immunosuppressive
- Moderate exercise lowers incidences of cold and flu, while heavy exercise loads increase them

Of course, some people can exercise for hours without over-exercising depending on their levels of fitness, modality, training experience, intensity, recovery, health, and age, and more so, it's impossible to give specific recommendations that fit every person. The key is to listen to your body. Rest days where little or no exercise occurs are also important.

If you do large volumes of exercise, particularly endurance exercise such as running, swimming, or cycling, also take care to eat a nutrient-dense diet, take nutritional supplements where appropriate, keep stress low, get plenty of sleep, and support recovery where you can. To ensure you aren't overdoing things, measure your heart rate variability (HRV) every morning upon waking. Over-exercising or illness will be reflected in your scores. A drop in your baseline HRV scores for a few days in a row indicates overtraining.

EAT PLENTY OF FIBER

You've likely been told to consume plenty of fiber in order to maintain a healthy digestive system, but there is much more to fiber than this! There are multiple types of fiber offering different biological and immune effects. Here's a quick rundown of some of the most important types of fiber and their immune benefits:

1. **Beta-glucans.** Beta-glucans are a type of soluble fiber that modulate the immune system by regulating the function of several types of immune cells, including macrophages, neutrophils, and lymphocytes. They have been used effectively to combat both viral and bacterial infections, combat cancer cells, and lower cholesterol and low-density lipoprotein levels. Beta-glucans are found in mushrooms and oats.

2. **Inulin.** Inulin is a soluble fiber that is an important prebiotic for certain strains of bacteria in the gut. It improves blood sugar levels and reduces gut inflammation. Sources of inulin include wheat, onion, bananas, garlic, and asparagus.

3. **Pectin.** Pectins are another type of soluble fiber that are a prebiotic for gut bacteria. They also lower blood sugar levels and improve blood lipid (cholesterol) markers. Apples, strawberries, citrus fruits, carrots, and potatoes are some of the best sources of pectin.

4. **Psyllium.** Psyllium is an insoluble fiber that is a prebiotic and softens stools, making them easier to pass. The fiber comes from the outer husk of the psyllium plant's seeds. You don't really find this fiber in foods; instead, you can get it as a powdered supplement.

5. **Lignin.** Lignin is an insoluble fiber that solidifies your stool and is believed to reduce risks of bowel cancer. Food sources of lignin

include whole-grain foods (wheat and corn bran), legumes (beans and peas), vegetables (green beans, cauliflower, zucchini), fruits (avocado, unripe bananas), and nuts and seeds (flaxseed).

6. **Resistant starch.** Resistant starch is similar to soluble fiber and lowers cholesterol, improves blood sugar levels, and may improve weight loss by reducing appetite. Oats, legumes, unripe bananas, beans, and cold potatoes are great sources of resistant starch.

Different fibers also feed different strains of bacteria. A recent study found that over twenty different types of fiber affect bacteria. Given that a diverse gut microbiota is critical to a healthy immune system, you need to consume a variety of different fibers. Both a lack of fiber and a lack of variety in fiber sources will compromise your gut microbiota and immunity. In general, men are recommended to consume 30–38 grams of fiber a day and women are recommended to consume 20–25 grams.

WRITE EXPRESSIVELY

Writing can be an effective tool with many health benefits. Expressive writing has been found to be particularly therapeutic, especially for the immune system. Expressive writing involves writing about events and circumstances that manifest intense and distressing emotions. Studies have found it improves:

- Levels of T lymphocyte immune cells
- Respiratory conditions such as asthma
- Immune response in HIV patients
- Autoimmune conditions such as rheumatoid arthritis
- Time taken to fall asleep when done before bed
- The healing of trauma, PTSD, and depression, which impair immune health
- Stress

It also has cathartic effects that support the release of distressing emotions that would otherwise suppress immune function. Researchers have concluded that expressive writing has similar benefits to working with a therapist. In order to gain from the healing and well-being benefits of expressive writing, it is important to write in detail about the event or circumstance affecting you, your thoughts and emotions relating to it, and, most importantly, any meaning you find in the situation. Simply venting emotions or describing the event without connecting to the emotions behind it is ineffective.

To benefit from this therapeutic activity you can either write about specific traumatic and emotional events when their pain surfaces or commit to regular journaling. Journaling is particularly effective since it can become a well-developed practice that enables you to process your day or week in a healthy way. It is recommended to write freely for about 15–20 minutes without editing your thoughts or words. It can also be helpful to focus on a specific theme for the day or week.

TAP YOURSELF TO STRONGER IMMUNITY

Emotional Freedom Technique (EFT), or Tapping, is an effective tool for reducing and even eliminating emotional stress. It is based on the idea that all negative emotions are the result of blockages within the body's energy pathways. It works in a similar way to acupuncture in Chinese medicine by unblocking these energy pathways, also known as meridians. It can be useful for releasing all types of emotional distress including fear, anxiety, anger, frustration, and depression. It is also useful in treating PTSD and even physical ailments.

In studies, EFT has been found to be an effective tool for lowering cortisol (the stress hormone), heart rate, and blood pressure, and for improving heart rate variability, a measure of nervous system stress. On an emotional and physical level, studies have shown its effectiveness in improving anxiety, depression, insomnia, respiratory issues, cravings, and PTSD. All of these improvements support immune health.

Studies examining EFT's effect on the immune system directly show that it lowers inflammation, improves expression of immune-related genes, increases immune cell levels, and upregulates immune antibodies such as SIgA, the main antibody found along the gut and respiratory tract. Studies also show it can be an effective tool for improving autoimmune conditions including psoriasis and fibromyalgia.

EFT is a simple technique you can learn and practice right at home. There are numerous online tutorials to walk you through EFT, although for specific conditions such as mental health or PTSD it is recommended to work with a trained EFT practitioner who can provide extra guidance.

CUT DOWN ON ALCOHOL

It likely comes as no surprise that alcohol consumption can seriously impair the immune system. Specifically, alcohol:

- Inhibits immune cell function
- Damages the mucosal lining of the digestive and respiratory systems, making them more porous and thus vulnerable to unwanted particles and microbes trying to enter the body
- Damages immune cells located on the mucosal lining of the digestive and respiratory tracts
- Kills healthy bacteria in the gut that aid in your immunity
- Elevates blood sugar levels, causing oxidative stress and inflammation
- Disrupts sleep, making you vulnerable to infection
- Causes pneumonia and autoimmune conditions (when consumed heavily)

It is not just chronic alcohol consumption that compromises immune function. Several studies have found that binge drinking (drinking excessive amounts in one session—usually five or more drinks for men and four or more drinks for women) impairs the body's natural capacity to heal itself.

The case for moderate alcohol consumption is sometimes made, on the basis that it lowers some inflammatory markers (c-reactive protein). The mechanisms behind this are not yet known. One likely explanation is that it is caused by other compounds found in alcoholic beverages, such as polyphenols and antioxidants found in red wine, not the alcohol. Of course, this doesn't eliminate the harmful effects of alcohol.

Health experts recommend drinking no more than twice a week or 2–3 drinks at a time. And since small amounts can still have detrimental effects, consuming as little alcohol as possible is best for optimal immune health.

MOVE MORE, MUCH MORE

A sedentary lifestyle causes huge damage to your health. Sedentary living includes a lack of exercise, excessive time spent sitting, and an overall lack of movement. Many people exercise several times a week but are sedentary the rest of it. Studies show sitting is as harmful as smoking, with eleven minutes of sitting as damaging as a single cigarette. Unfortunately, regular exercise does little to mitigate these harmful effects. Additionally:

- Sedentary behavior causes inflammation, while physical activity reduces it
- Sedentary behavior reduces the response of immune cells to infection
- Movement elevates levels of adenosine, which regulates immune function, reduces inflammation, and makes deep sleep possible
- Inactivity causes a buildup of toxins that harm the mitochondria in your cells, which weakens your immune health
- Sedentary behavior is linked to obesity, depression, diabetes, insulin resistance, cardiovascular disease, and other conditions of chronic inflammation and immune impairment

There's no agreed-upon guideline for how much non-exercise physical activity you need, but few get enough. Ten thousand steps is touted as the magic number, but it's not enough. For the average person that's just ninety minutes of walking—less than 10 percent of your waking day. Most people don't get this number of steps in, so it's a good place to start but is far from optimal.

Do whatever you can to move more, ideally at least three hours a day (including exercise). Use public transport and drive only when necessary, park or get on/off transport farther from your destination, use a standing desk, conduct walking meetings, and, most importantly, change your attitude toward one of seeking opportunities to move rather than avoiding them.

EAT YOUR FISH

The health benefits of omega-3 fatty acids are well researched. They provide structural and anti-inflammatory benefits. There are three main types of omega-3: eicosapentaenoic acid (EPA), docosahexaenoic acid (DHA), and alpha-linolenic acid (ALA). EPA and DHA are sourced mainly from animals and fish products, while ALA is sourced from plant products. EPA provides mainly anti-inflammatory effects, and DHA provides anti-inflammatory and structural benefits (predominantly the formation of cell membranes and the brain).

The anti-inflammatory effects of omega-3s include:

- Reduced pro-inflammatory cytokines (immune messengers)
- Reduced eicosanoids (signaling molecules that regulate inflammation)
- Reduced inflammatory markers (e.g., c-reactive protein)
- Reduced gene expression of inflammatory compounds
- Production of resolvins, which have anti-inflammatory effects

Increasing omega-3 intake improves several inflammatory conditions including depression, anxiety, Alzheimer's, asthma, and autoimmune conditions (lupus, psoriasis, rheumatoid arthritis, inflammatory bowel disease, metabolic syndrome, heart disease, type 1 diabetes, etc.).

While there is some evidence of changes in activity within some immune cells, the effect of omega-3s on immune cells appears to be largely inhibitory. The resolvins that they produce also have some antimicrobial effects. Omega-3s are also linked to better sleep and mood, both of which will help to improve immune health.

Because of their strong anti-inflammatory effects, it is best to avoid the consumption of high amounts of omega-3s during the initial stages of an acute infection (e.g., common cold or flu) when a strong immune response is preferable. Recommended intakes of DHA and EPA combined is 200–500 milligrams per day. The upper limit for combined intake is 3,000 milligrams. At least one third of your daily intake should come from food, especially oily fish, which are the richest animal sources of omega-3s. It is recommended to consume at least two 3.5-ounce servings of oily fish a week to get sufficient omega-3s.

Many fish oils are high in heavy metals (such as mercury) and are easily oxidized, so be sure to do some research into the quality of a fish oil before purchasing. At a minimum it should be free from heavy metals, cold pressed, and contain antioxidants to protect it from oxidization. Fish oil capsules are likely to be better protected from metals and oxidization. Always store capsules in the refrigerator.

FIND YOUR CREATIVE OUTLET

Studies show that creativity is an effective vehicle for improving immune health. It has been explored through various forms of therapy to improve mental, emotional, and immune well-being.

In general, studies exploring creative expression have found that it can:

- Increase immune cell production
- Improve mental health by lowering depression, anxiety, and stress, and healing trauma
- Lower cortisol (the stress hormone)
- Lower inflammation
- Improve mood
- Build self-esteem
- Improve immune-related conditions

Not all benefits are equal across all forms of creativity, however. For example, singing is best for stimulating and strengthening the parasympathetic nervous system, while dance is best to get the lymphatic system flowing, and expressive writing is great for processing emotional stress. Common modalities for creative expression include art and crafts, dance, music, singing, cooking, and writing. The form your own creative expression takes is not important; what *is* important is that you enjoy it.

Some people pursue creative expression as their career. From a health perspective this may not always be beneficial, as egocentric needs such as recognition or money are more likely to overpower the healing power and fun of creative expression. When that happens, some benefits associated with creativity may be lost. Famous poet Oscar Wilde once said, "All art is quite useless," meaning art exists for the joy of art, and for no other use.

MIX WITH MICROBES

Microorganisms play crucial roles in the development of your immune system. Many people think of microbes as the enemy of the immune system, but they are actually its best friend.

During the early stages of life, microorganisms in your external and internal environment (your microbiota) teach and hone the immune system so that it learns to regulate itself. An unregulated immune system becomes hypersensitive and over-reactive.

As society has developed, it has introduced sanitation, clean water, garbage collection, pasteurization, smaller families, a move from rural environments, antibiotics, and antibacterial cleaning products. These advancements have dramatically changed the terrain that shapes the way the immune system develops. It is no longer exposed to the vast and diverse microbial environment it once was.

These changes are believed to be behind much of the rise in allergies and autoimmunity of recent decades. Fifty million Americans have an autoimmune condition and 12.5 percent of children in the US have eczema. The risk of developing an allergy or autoimmune condition, either in childhood or later life, is dramatically increased with low exposure, especially at a young age. This leads to a hypersensitive and overactive immune system that has less capacity to combat new infections.

If you want to develop a healthy, well-balanced immune system then you must be exposed to various sources of microorganisms. This is essential to the diversity of your microbiota and your immune system's ability to self-regulate.

Exposure during the first few years of life, especially the first few months, is critical. Animals (pets, farm animals, etc.), natural environments, and physical contact with others will provide this exposure that is needed for the development of the immune system and microbiota.

FORGIVE YOURSELF

One of the best things you can do for your health and happiness is forgive. And while it is important to forgive others, the most important person you must forgive is yourself.

Directing your resentments, frustrations, and anger inward in the forms of self-hate, self-doubt, self-criticism, and shame is especially damaging, as you are both sending and receiving these toxic emotions—giving you a double dose. Anger, resentment, shame, and similar emotions trigger a stress response in the body, shutting down the immune system.

The job of your immune system is to protect you from harm, so what if that harm is coming from yourself?

It's common to find those with autoimmune conditions, in which the immune system sees the body as the enemy, to have tendencies toward self-loathing, lacking in self-acceptance. In such situations it is theorized that the body is mirroring the psyche. The mind-body connection really is *that* strong. For example, self-hatred can arise from childhood abuse, as it's during early childhood that you form your relationship with yourself, based on how you are treated, especially by your caregivers. Abuse often teaches you that you are bad and deserve punishment. It's therefore no surprise that research shows that the majority of those with autoimmunity experienced childhood trauma.

Self-forgiveness is an especially powerful medicine. It helps release a great deal of toxic emotions and stress, enabling your immune system to work in healthier ways. Practice directing greater forgiveness and compassion toward yourself now. You can journal out what you are upset about and why you deserve to be forgiven, write a letter of forgiveness to yourself, or even recite a self-forgiving mantra until the words take a deeper hold. Author and speaker Colin Tipping also developed a useful process on self-forgiveness that you can learn more about online.

USE COCONUT OIL

Coconut oil has been established as a health food for years, but do its health benefits aid the immune system? Without a doubt—yes!

Interestingly, some aspects of coconut oil make it similar to a mother's milk, which plays a critical role in building an infant's immune system. Lauric acid makes up 20 percent of the content in mother's milk, while coconut oil is 50 percent lauric acid—making it the closest food in nature to mother's milk in terms of lauric acid content.

The lauric acid found in coconut oil has strong antimicrobial properties. It also contains caprylic acid, another powerful antimicrobial. Many studies have found coconut oil to be effective at killing harmful bacteria, viruses, and fungi. It has also been used effectively to promote wound healing and tackle skin and oral infections.

Coconut oil is the richest food source of medium-chain triglycerides (MCTs). MCTs increase energy, reduce appetite, increase metabolism, and stimulate fat burning. By stimulating metabolism and aiding fat burning, MCTs also help lower inflammation. Coconut oil also aids blood sugar regulation and provides antioxidant and anti-inflammatory benefits, further enhancing its immune effects.

Recent studies have shown that coconut oil helps improve the microbiota in the gut and regulates the immune system. A 2020 study found that it regulates the immune system by regulating immune cytokines and immune cells (neutrophils and lymphocytes).

When consuming coconut oil, make sure it is cold-pressed, virgin coconut oil. Coconut oil can be used in cooking (avoid cooking with it at high temperatures), added to smoothies, applied as a moisturizer or makeup remover, or consumed as a supplement. Typically, 1–2 tablespoons a day are recommended for consumption.

CONSIDER STARVING A COLD *AND* A FEVER

Have you ever heard the expression "Feed a cold, starve a fever"? It is thought that this came about because eating helps the body to generate heat during a cold, while starving a fever could help reduce body temperature. While science suggests this is a half-truth at best, there are immune benefits to "starving a fever" that may support the fight against infection. "Starving," or "fasting," can trigger both:

1. **Apoptosis:** Cell suicide
2. **Autophagy:** The mechanism by which the body breaks down cells and reuses the material to make new cells

All viruses and many types of bacteria are intracellular, meaning that they invade your cells. Viruses do this to hijack cell DNA so that they can replicate, and bacteria do so to feed and protect themselves from the immune system. One mechanism used by the body to fight these invaders is apoptosis. The cell's death exposes the pathogen to specialized immune cells that target and engulf them. Autophagy is another cell response that works a little differently. During autophagy, parts of the invading microbe are sent to the lysosomes (the cell's digestive system) for destruction.

Both these mechanisms explain the instinct to avoid food when ill. It's a natural response to infection, so why interrupt it? Evolutionarily speaking, a lack of appetite also means that you are less likely to wander off to find food, allowing you to rest, heal, and contain the spread of infection, thereby protecting your tribe. It also starves the harmful microbes of zinc and iron that would otherwise support their growth.

The common cold and flu are caused by viruses, so it makes sense that they trigger a loss of appetite. Bacterial infections only occur during a cold or flu because the weakening of the immune system has left you vulnerable to a secondary (bacterial) infection. Some bacteria are extracellular, so fasting would provide little advantage against them. It may well be that when you are ill with an appetite you are infected with an extracellular bacterial infection.

The disadvantage of fasting is that it reduces intake of compounds, nutrients, and calories that may strengthen the immune system, which is why fasting when sick isn't always best. If you are in good health, going a day or two without food is unlikely to weaken you. If your loss of appetite lasts longer than 2–3 days it may help to eat.

Nature programmed your body to instinctively understand what is needed. It knows when the infection is viral and when the infection is an intracellular or extracellular bacteria, so trust your innate responses. If you feel hungry and need to eat, eat. And if you have no appetite don't force it, as you may interrupt your intelligent immune response and hinder your recovery.

CLEAN YOUR AIR

One of the main roles of the immune system is to protect your body from anything it views as harmful. This includes viruses, bacteria, and parasites, but also allergens. The most common source of immune irritants beyond microbes are man-made substances or natural compounds at artificially high levels (e.g., artificial chemicals and heavy metals). These can provoke, suppress, or damage the immune system.

These substances can make it into your body from toxic outdoor and indoor air via your respiratory system. While there is little you can personally do about outdoor air, you can take action to improve the air quality in your home.

Removing as many chemical toxins from your living spaces as possible is a good place to start. Some of these chemicals get into the air and damage the lining of the lungs (home to part of the immune system) and can cause inflammation, for example asthma. Others simply add to the carnival of unnatural chemicals floating around your body, stressing and damaging your cells and organs.

Using chemical-based cleaning products just once a week has been found to cause lung damage equal to smoking twenty cigarettes a day. The most researched airborne compounds are volatile organic compounds (VOCs). These are used in various products including cleaning products, insect repellents, air fresheners, glues, paints, varnishes, and building materials. They irritate the eyes, nose, and throat, and cause fatigue, headache, and cancer.

Aside from eliminating toxic chemicals, it is recommended to improve the quality of your indoor air by regularly opening windows, using high-efficiency particulate air (HEPA) filters, and decorating with house plants that are proven to clean the air (e.g., peace lilies, spider plants, and rubber plants).

REDUCE CHEMICALS IN YOUR FOOD

Unless you are consuming a diet of mainly organic whole natural foods, you are likely to be bombarding your body and immune system with harmful unnatural substances. Here's one main reason why: food chemicals.

Food chemicals are used a lot in processed foods in order to increase shelf life or to increase sensory appeal via taste, smell, look, or texture. Some food chemicals are even used to hijack your brain so that you crave the food more. Unfortunately, consuming these foods comes at a heavy cost to your health. Common food chemicals that impair immune function include aspartame, MSG (monosodium glutamate), Sunset Yellow FCF, tartrazine, sodium sulfite, sodium benzoate, cinnamaldehyde, propionic acid, carrageenan, and emulsifiers. These food chemicals can affect the immune system in a host of ways, including damaging some types of immune cells, inhibiting the release of both inflammatory and inhibitory cytokines (immune messengers), triggering allergic response, making the immune system hypersensitive, and harming the microbiota in the gut.

You can do much to limit your intake of these harmful chemicals by eating a whole food diet, making your own meals, and eating organic.

TAKE PRECAUTIONS WHEN FLYING

Your risk of developing an infection increases significantly when traveling, particularly flying.

Traveling is very stressful on the body, especially when traveling across time zones. It usually involves disrupting regular sleep times because of travel, extra stress from rushing to get to the airport on time, and environmental changes including changes in air pressure and temperature, all of which lower immunity.

When on the plane you are also exposed to high concentrations of electromagnetic stress from the plane's electrical wiring, electronics, TV screens in headrests, Wi-Fi, and countless personal mobile devices. This is made worse because planes are made of material designed to keep radiation (from the sun) out, but in doing so they also keep electromagnetic radiation in. You are also exposed to humidity that is 10 percent lower than normal, which can dry out the mucus found in the nose and throat that is there to trap and help defend you against pathogens.

Once you reach your destination you may also be exposed to alien microbes—especially if you traveled abroad—from new foods, water, and airborne pathogens. And in some cases you may have moved across time zones, disrupting circadian rhythm and sleep patterns. This is all a recipe for weakened immunity and exposure to new microbes that you have no immunity to.

Luckily there are many choices you can make to mitigate infection risk when flying:

- Drink plenty of water before, during, and after flying
- Eat a high-quality diet in the days before, during, and after travel—emphasizing immune-boosting plant foods
- Minimize the intake of alcohol, sugar, and caffeine, which suppress immune activity, in the twenty-four hours before and after flying

- Support immunity with supplements beginning twenty-four hours before traveling and ending 24–48 hours after your return, including any combination of:
    - Vitamin C
    - Zinc
    - High dose probiotic
    - Glutathione
    - Melatonin (if jet lag is an issue)
    - Echinacea
    - *Panax* (Asian) *ginseng*
    - Ashwagandha
- Connect to the earth by grounding for at least thirty minutes upon arrival (this neutralizes the accumulation of positive ions from the flight)
- Minimize jet lag when traveling east; avoid staying up late and get into a dark environment with minimal (blue) light when the sun sets, get lots of natural light in the first half of the day, and avoid sleeping in
- Minimize jet lag when traveling west by getting plenty of natural light in the hours before sunset to delay tiredness
- Gently adjust timing of your sleep, eating, light, and exercise habits toward your new destination in the forty-eight hours before a long flight
- Use hand sanitizers and wipes—especially on food trays, seat pockets, touchscreens, inflight magazines, and the restroom—to reduce exposure to unwanted microbes

Practice as many of these precautions as possible whenever flying: Your immune health will thank you!

FILTER YOUR WATER

None of the water you drink is likely to be very pure, as it contains compounds that disrupt the way your immune system and body work. Compounds found in your water supply can include:

1. **Heavy metals.** These find their way into your water supply because the water pipes running from the water company to your home may be very old (particularly if your home is old) and leach metals such as lead, nickel, and copper into the water. Heavy metals may also come from agricultural chemical runoff from farming. These metals can damage organs and glands of the immune system as well as inhibit or stimulate inappropriate immune responses.

2. **Chlorine.** Chlorine is used to kill harmful microbes that would otherwise contaminate the water. While this is helpful, you don't want the chlorine in your body, as it can also harm microbes that support immune health.

3. **Pharmaceutical drug residues.** When consumed, drugs are not completely absorbed into the body and significant quantities end up flushed down the toilet. These are not filtered out during water treatment, meaning some of them may be in the water you are drinking and using in your home. Even at small amounts, they can build up and cause problems in the body, potentially harming the immune system.

4. **Agricultural chemical residues.** These chemicals run off farms and into the rivers and lakes, eventually ending up in your water supply. These are not filtered by water companies, meaning they can make it into your home water and cause problems.

To avoid these potential dangers to your immune system, filter your water—be it the water you drink, cook with, or wash in—using a combination of filters such as:

- Whole house filtration system
- Shower filter
- Reverse osmosis
- Gravitational filter
- Water bottle filter

Cleaner water means a happier immune system!

CHANGE YOUR CLEANING AND PERSONAL CARE PRODUCTS

Man-made chemicals and/or unnatural levels of natural compounds have been shown to cause significant damage to health and well-being. They can disrupt the immune system in many ways, contributing to immune-related problems including fatigue, inflammation, autoimmune conditions, and more.

Some chemical toxins are proven to damage the lungs, nose, eyes, and throat (which house immune cells); disrupt the microbiota in the gut, which plays important roles in immunity; and damage the mitochondria in cells that have a very powerful influence on the immune system. Some chemicals are also known to damage the brain and nervous system (neurotoxins) and the endocrine system (endotoxins), which both play important roles in regulating the immune system. Additionally, there are chemicals known to damage the way immune cells work.

Although these chemicals come from many sources, some of the main sources are cleaning and personal care products. These include everything from toilet, window, oven, floor, and surface cleaners to your makeup, toothpaste, soaps, and perfumes. Chemicals found in these products can get into your body through your skin, the air you breathe, and chemical residues on cutlery and dishes washed in these substances. Some of these products, like makeup, also contain heavy metals, which can accumulate and cause significant damage to your organs.

The greater your exposure to these chemicals, the worse your health and the more affected your immune system is likely to be. Instead of using commercial products, use natural and plant-based alternatives that do not have such harmful effects. You can either buy natural products or make your own using very simple ingredients. Get more information, and easy recipes, online.

TURN OFF YOUR TV

The connection between TV and your immune system may not be immediately obvious, but for many reasons, cutting down your viewing hours can provide benefits to your immunity.

The first problem with TV is that it distracts you from other, healthier activities. TV shows can be addictive and encourage poor sleep habits and a sedentary lifestyle. TV keeps you indoors and away from the beneficial effects of sunlight, fresh air, and nature. It discourages you from socializing with friends and family who nourish your immune system. Prolonged TV viewing is also linked to antisocial behavior in children, type 2 diabetes, cardiovascular disease, and obesity, all of which weaken immunity.

The second major problem with TV is its detrimental psychological and emotional effects. News channels constantly stream messages of negativity, giving you endless reasons to feel fearful, depressed, and isolated. TV shows and movies reinforce unrealistic ideals and values about things like romance, success, and money that promote feelings of inadequacy and low self-esteem. They typically glorify money, sex, power, and materialism as the path to happiness. TV commercials also reinforce these messages and bombard you with marketing messages that attempt to push you into buying things that you don't need. The accumulated effect of all these messages is a mindset that fosters feelings of fear, anxiety, depression, anger, loneliness, and hate—all immunosuppressive emotions.

This isn't to say that all TV is bad, but to truly enjoy the health and happiness that you desire, you must be selective about what and how much you watch. Are the shows and movies you're watching supporting the development of a healthy, positive mind and body, or are they taking that away? Are the core messages behind what you watch consistent with how you wish to think, feel, and experience life? If not, you may want to rethink your viewing habits.

CONSUME FOOD OF THE GODS

Chocolate is often referred to as the "food of the gods," with good reason. Studies show that it contains many beneficial properties. Those most relevant to immune health include:

- Regulating inflammatory immune messengers (cytokines) and cells and improving inflammatory conditions such as hypertension and atherosclerosis
- Improving insulin resistance and metabolic health, which improves conditions such as diabetes, obesity, and metabolic syndrome
- Improving asthma through the helpful compounds theobromine and theophylline
- Combating oxidative stress, lowering inflammation, and supporting healthy gut microbiota via it's high polyphenol content
- Boosting mood and regulating immune function via it's high tryptophan (the precursor to serotonin) content
- Enhancing immune antibody response to the flu vaccine when consumed regularly
- Boosting immune health via iron and magnesium

Most chocolate and cocoa powder products are low quality and laden with harmful substances such as sugar. For optimal immune health benefits enjoy forms that are minimally processed. Cocoa is produced from cacao, making it inferior since it's gone through extra processing, destroying many nutrients. The healthiest forms of cacao include:

- Cacao nibs
- Raw cacao powder
- Dark chocolate low in sugar, over 80 percent cacao solids and with minimal other ingredients
- Ceremonial-grade cacao

GET BLUE LIGHT AT THE RIGHT TIMES

The depth of sunlight's effect on your immune system is seen when we examine the different wavelengths of light emitted by the sun. One of the most influential lights on the immune system is blue light.

Blue light can have positive effects on your immune defenses depending upon the timing, intensity, duration, and other factors affecting exposure. Blue light exposure during daylight hours suppresses melatonin and regulates the circadian rhythm, which is good news for your daytime immunity. It has also been found to have antibacterial effects and improve the motility of immune T lymphocytes cells, which simply means that it energizes them so that they are more mobile and function better. On the psychological side, blue light helps reduce depression, which is known to suppress immune function.

On the other hand, blue light, particularly that used by artificial lights and TV and phone screens, should be avoided at night, as it can disrupt sleep, circadian rhythm, and melatonin production. Overall, your blue light exposure should come from natural sources, aka sunlight, whenever possible, as some of the negative biological effects of blue light can in part be mitigated by the effects of other wavelengths, mainly red and infrared wavelengths.

VISIT A SAUNA

Saunas have been used for thousands of years by cultures all around the world, from shamanic sweat lodges to traditional Finnish saunas. And in recent years, scientists have validated this ancient practice for health improvement.

Regular sauna use:

- Reduces the incidences of colds and flu
- Increases several types of immune cells in the short and longer term
- Improves stress (lowers levels of the stress hormone cortisol), anxiety, and depression
- Elevates mood
- Improves autoimmune (chronic fatigue syndrome and rheumatoid arthritis) and chronic inflammatory (cardiovascular, lung and brain diseases) conditions
- Detoxifies the body, through sweating, of chemical toxins and heavy metals (e.g., lead, arsenic, and thiuram) that disrupt immune function (infrared saunas only)
- Improves sleep when used a couple of hours before bed
- Increases autophagy (the recycling and replacement of redundant immune and other cells)

Saunas provide these immune benefits because they emit infrared light, which provides many immune benefits including healing, energy, immune-cell-generating, anti-inflammatory, and antioxidant benefits. They also produce heat, which raises core body temperature by a few degrees, imitating the effects of a fever, a natural response to some infections. This "fake" fever activates the immune response responsible for fighting microbes and the immune system's memory. The heat also activates heat shock proteins, which trigger an immune response and have antimicrobial and inflammatory effects.

To optimize long-term benefits, aim to use a sauna four or more days a week. (Occasional use will still produce short-term benefits.) If you are new to saunas, begin with 5–15 minutes per session and increase use over time. Use Finnish saunas for up to one hour and forty minutes for infrared saunas. Make sure you are fully hydrated before and after using a sauna. If you are pregnant or have a cardiovascular condition seek your doctor's advice first.

COMBAT COLDS AND SEASONAL ALLERGIES WITH ASTRAGALUS

Astragalus is a root used in Chinese medicine and is often taken to combat the common cold and other upper respiratory infections. Astragalus contains compounds known to strengthen immunity, including:

- Polysaccharides, which lower levels of pro-inflammatory cytokines
- Flavonoids, which lower oxidative stress levels
- Saponins, which boost immune function and may improve cholesterol levels
- Immune-supporting minerals zinc, selenium, and sometimes copper

Astragalus has also been found to:

- Increase levels of immune cells
- Increase thymus and spleen function
- Improve the common cold and seasonal allergies (e.g., hay fever)
- Provide antibacterial and antiviral effects
- Regulate blood sugar levels and improve diabetes
- Improve anemia
- Possibly have anticancer effects
- Boost the effectiveness of several types of vaccines (in animal tests only)
- Improve lung function and asthma

It can be extracted into various forms such as capsules, powders, teas, and tinctures. Typical dosages are 1–4 grams of the dried root, up to 1 gram three times a day of capsules, or up to 6 milliliters three times a day of a tincture. As tea, 9–15 grams are typically taken. Astragalus is not recommended for use by anyone who has a Th1-related autoimmune condition or is taking immunosuppressive drugs.

UNDERSTAND THE SCHUMANN RESONANCE

The Schumann resonance (SR) is the name for the frequencies of the earth's electromagnetic field. The earth doesn't have just one frequency, but a mix of eight that operate within a range of 3–60 Hz (7.83 Hz is the base frequency that people are most familiar with). It occasionally exceeds this range.

This electromagnetic charge comes from the sun, which emits electromagnetic plasma (radiation)—in the form of solar flares and solar wind—that takes anywhere from eight minutes to several days to reach the earth. Once it reaches the earth this charge accumulates within the earth's ionosphere and magnetosphere and is discharged to the earth via lightning, which strikes the earth fifty(!) times every second. As lightning strikes the earth, electromagnetic waves are dispersed, creating the SR within the cavity between the earth and the ionosphere. The different frequencies of this SR change in intensity in accordance with changes in the ionosphere and solar activity.

During intense periods of solar activity hitting the earth, geomagnetic storms are created that raise the frequencies of SR. Studies show that during these periods of SR elevation, similar elevations are seen within the frequencies of the brain and nervous system (which operate at similar frequencies), impacting human health and behavior. This resonance effect has been called "magnetoreception" by scientists.

Studies have found that magnetoreception causes changes in blood pressure, heart rate, and heart rate variability. During these periods cardiac incidences, depression, suicide, traffic accidents, and crime are measurably increased in the areas of the world affected. Effects may also be seen before/after the storm, as the electromagnetic changes will start beforehand and it can take days or even weeks for a person's nervous system to return to normal. Sensitivity to SR elevation varies between individuals and it is believed that about 10–15 percent of the world population is impacted by geomagnetic-related health problems.

Because of the strong relationship between the nervous system and the immune system, these changes have implications for your immune health too, and understanding the Schumann resonance and potential changes to it enables you to predict when you are most at risk of infection. You can learn more about these changes and track them at www.heartmath.org/gci/gcms/.

A regular practice of grounding to the earth (e.g., walking/standing barefoot outside) will neutralize any extra nervous system excitability brought on by SR elevation. Pulsed electromagnetic field therapy may also help, as well as a diet rich in antioxidants. Check out more information on pulsed electromagnetic field therapy online.

DRINK GREEN TEA

The health benefits of green tea are well established, especially for enhancing immune function. (Keep in mind green tea can be harmful to those with autoimmunity, so talk to your doctor first before drinking green tea if autoimmune.)

Many of the beneficial properties of green tea are due to its polyphenol (beneficial compounds unique to plants) content, particularly its EGCG (epigallocatechin gallate) content. EGCG is a powerful antioxidant that neutralizes free radicals, is antibacterial, and helps to prevent inflammation. Green tea is also a rich source of L-theanine, an amino acid with immune benefits. L-theanine increases levels of a specialized lymphocyte immune cell, reduces anxiety, and has antiviral effects.

Studies show that green tea is antiviral and provides a three-fold protection against the flu. Additionally, it helps immune-related conditions, protects against cancer, and improves cardiovascular disease, diabetes, and blood sugar regulation.

You can strengthen your immune health every day by drinking green tea or using a green tea supplement for a more concentrated dose. A popular form of green tea is matcha green tea, which has ten times higher levels of EGCG.

It is not recommended to consume more than 400 micrograms of EGCG per day. Because of the caffeine content of green tea (30–50 micrograms), it is recommended to consume no more than 100 micrograms of caffeine daily.

CRY IT OUT

Although attitudes are changing, for a long time, crying has been viewed by many as a sign of weakness—which has meant that people have missed out on its therapeutic benefits. These include stress release, healing, and stronger immunity. It is true: Despite the temptation to hold back our tears, research tells us that we are better off allowing things to flow.

The ingredients of our tears vary. Basal or continuous tears are released every time we blink and contain water, fats, and proteins that moisten and protect the eye. Reflex tears contain similar ingredients and are released when we get something in our eye. Emotional tears are released during periods of emotional distress. They contain a mix of toxins and hormones including:

- Potassium and manganese, which help lower blood pressure and cholesterol
- Prolactin, which lowers stress and strengthens immunity
- Oxytocin, which eases physical and emotional pain and provides a sense of calmness
- A potent bacteria-fighting protein called lysozyme, thought to protect us from infection when we are most stressed and vulnerable

Aside from the ingredients of tears, crying deepens your breathing and activates the parasympathetic nervous system, which lowers stress and cortisol (the stress hormone) levels while strengthening your immune response. In many cases crying also brings about social support and compassion from others, which further strengthens immunity.

In one study, 88.8 percent of those surveyed reported that crying helped them to improve mood. Meanwhile, suppressing tears and emotions increases stress and damages emotional and immune well-being. The stress benefits of crying have even led to "crying clubs," called "rui-katsu," in Japan, where members come together for group crying therapy.

PAY IT FORWARD

Being kind to others is not as selfless as you might think—at least in terms of your immune well-being. Research shows that kindness (simply putting someone else's needs ahead of your own) bolsters your immunity.

Kindness increases levels of oxytocin (the love and bonding hormone) and serotonin (the happiness hormone). Both regulate the immune system and lower depression. Oxytocin also lowers stress hormones, inflammation, and oxidative stress. Kindness also increases self-esteem, proven to strengthen immunity, by encouraging you to see the good and value in yourself. Further, meditating on kind thoughts and feelings (such as a loving kindness meditation) increases heart rate variability, known to improve immune function.

And kindness doesn't just benefit you. It creates a feeling of well-being and improved immunity in the receiver and anyone witnessing the act as well. How? It's all thanks to mirror neurons in the brain, which allow you to imitate the language, facial expressions, and emotions of those you observe. When you demonstrate kindness, everyone around you benefits from the same immune effects. This is known as the "Mother Teresa Effect," a term originating from a study that measured the immune system effects of watching a video of Mother Teresa carrying out acts of kindness. Elevations in the immune antibody SIgA were observed in viewers both during and immediately following the video, indicating stronger immunity. Research also shows that witnessing a kind act increases your desire to pay it forward and be kind to others.

Kindness extended, received, or observed is great for the immune system. Through one simple act of kindness you can create a ripple effect that benefits the immunity of thousands. Be kind to others and you strengthen everyone's immune health.

CONSIDER LACTOFERRIN

Lactoferrin is a glycoprotein that has a number of health benefits, including those involved in immunity. It is naturally found in the human body wherever you find the mucosal lining (e.g., breast milk, saliva, tears, semen, vaginal fluid, lungs, nose, digestive juices, and urine). It plays important roles in the development of an infant's immune and digestive system. Supplementing with lactoferrin can support immunity because it:

- Stimulates the action of immune cells including natural killer cells, neutrophils, macrophages, and some other lymphocytes
- Has anti-inflammatory effects
- May help reduce asthma and allergies
- Binds with iron (essential to immune health) and increases its absorption in the gut
- Prevents harmful bacteria from using iron in the blood for their growth, which makes it a powerful antibacterial agent
- Has antioxidant benefits (because it binds with iron), helping to lower oxidative stress
- Has antiviral, antifungal, and antiparasitic properties
- Can help reduce obesity and insulin resistance, which cause chronic inflammation
- Has anticancer effects

Research into lactoferrin supplementation is in its infancy so much is still unknown. It is safe to supplement, however, and studies have typically used dosages of 300–600 milligrams, sometimes as high as 3,000 milligrams. Doses above 1,100 milligrams per day may cause digestive issues.

It is likely to be particularly beneficial to anyone who has a bacterial infection, is frequently ill, and/or is iron deficient. Lactoferrin is sourced from either cow's milk or genetically modified rice, so check the source when supplementing with it in order to ensure that it is in a form acceptable to you.

SUPPORT YOUR MICROBIOTA

The microscopic organisms of your gut microbiota play important roles in your immune health. They help combat pathogenic microbes, regulate the immune system, produce beneficial nutrients (short-chain fatty acids, vitamin B12, vitmain K, thiamine, and riboflavin), and help train your immune system so that it produces healthy balanced responses against invaders. Maintaining a healthy balance between beneficial (85 percent) and harmful (15 percent) bacteria, a high diversity of strains, and volume of bacteria in your microbiota is essential to performing these roles. Low levels of both diversity and volume have been linked to many ill health conditions and diseases affecting areas such as the gut and brain; restoring levels significantly improves these conditions.

Of all the ways to maintain a healthy microbiota balance, the most important is your diet. Some foods will damage the delicate balance of your microbiota in your gut, while others will help increase both the diversity and numbers found in the gut.

Foods that are good for your microbiota health include:

- Foods rich in prebiotic fibers, such as legumes, onions, garlic, asparagus, oats, bananas, leeks, seaweed, apples, cashew nuts, coconut meal, cocoa powder, chicory root, cabbage, berries, sweet potato, and artichokes
- Foods rich in resistant starch, such as white potatoes, sweet potatoes, or rice that have been cooked then cooled; white beans; lentils; and green bananas
- Foods rich in polyphenols, such as berries, cocoa powder, dark chocolate, green or black tea, blackcurrants, cherries, cloves, nuts (especially hazelnuts and pecans), artichokes, chicory, red onion, spinach, and white or black beans

- Fermented foods such as kombucha, sauerkraut, kefir, kimchi, tempeh, yogurt (unflavored, natural, or Greek), and fermented vegetables

Foods that are bad for your microbiota health include:

- Alcohol
- Refined carbohydrates and sugar
- Processed foods
- Chlorinated water

Aside from improving your diet, other proven ways to improve your microbiota include reducing stress, spending time in nature and with animals (e.g., pets), physical contact with other people, exercising, getting good sleep, kicking a smoking habit, and avoiding antibiotics.

REDUCE YOUR EXPOSURE TO HEAVY METALS

Overexposure to heavy metals has damaging effects on almost every system, organ, and gland. They can inhibit or stimulate the immune system, impairing its ability to do its job. Heavy metal toxicity has been linked to allergies, autoimmunity, cancer, and various inflammatory diseases. Some metals are needed in small quantities for good health (copper, zinc, and iron) while others aren't needed at all (aluminum, lead, and mercury).

The effect of a heavy metal is determined by its form, level of exposure, rate of absorption or elimination, and health status. Some metals accumulate in the body, making long-term, low-level exposure problematic. While it's impossible to eliminate heavy metal exposure completely, you can eliminate unnecessary exposure to improve your health. Here is a list of the most common sources of heavy metals:

- **Mercury:** Mercury amalgams, fish, shellfish, some vaccines (thimerosal)
- **Aluminum:** Aluminum foil, cookware, tap water, pharmaceuticals, pesticides, cigarettes
- **Arsenic:** Pesticides, cigarettes
- **Copper:** Contraceptive pills, cookware, tap water (from water pipes), shellfish
- **Cadmium:** Cigarettes, tap water, instant coffee, paint, pesticides, large fish, rice
- **Iron:** Tap water, cookware
- **Lead:** Tap water, cosmetics (lipstick), diesel, cigarette smoke

To help reduce exposure from seafood, consume wild sources and small fish (mackerel, sardines, and shellfish).

If you have mercury fillings only get them removed if they are leaching mercury into your system. Otherwise you risk leaching them into the body upon removal. Talk to a dental professional practicing holistic dentistry to find out the best option for you.

Detoxifying heavy metals can be done using appropriate chelating substances with the help of a trained professional. Additionally, you can help your body to naturally and safely detoxify heavy metals by using infrared saunas, drinking plenty of water, and consuming chlorella, spirulina, garlic, glutathione, and probiotics.

DRINK CEREMONIAL CACAO

Cacao and cocoa have many immune health benefits including anti-inflammatory, antioxidant, microbiota, and immune-modulating effects. But the two are not equally beneficial. Cocoa originates from the cacao bean and is used to make most chocolate products. Through heavy processing and manufacturing many of cacao's beneficial nutrients and compounds are lost. In addition, most chocolate products are then mixed with sugar, unhealthy fats, and food chemicals, making them unhealthy. Cacao powder is healthier, although it still goes through much processing and many of its natural fiber and nutritious fats (cacao butter) are removed, making it much less nutritious.

The purest and healthiest form of cacao is ceremonial-grade cacao. This is produced using traditional processes that are gentle and maintain cacao's beneficial nutrients and compounds. Although most studies use cocoa, significant health benefits are still observed, and ceremonial-grade cacao is likely to provide vastly greater benefits than cocoa.

While it tastes similar to chocolate, ceremonial-grade cacao is much more bitter. It is called "ceremonial" because it has been used by traditional and ancient cultures across Mesoamerica for thousands of years during ceremonies to enrich the mind, body, and soul. According to these traditions, ceremonial-grade cacao offers many healing and energetic benefits that go beyond the physical body.

Aside from its immune benefits, it has powerful properties that can help open up the heart. Opening the heart and heart-centered emotions (love, gratitude, and compassion) provide your immune health with a huge boost as they lower inflammation and stress, improve mental well-being, and increase levels of immune cells and oxytocin.

Because cacao contains caffeine (an average of 25 milligrams per cup, although it varies greatly depending on the product) be careful of total caffeine intake from all sources across the day.

HEAL PTSD

Traumatic events often stay with us for years—even decades. Post-Traumatic Stress Disorder (PTSD) is the name given when an event has left an obvious emotional scar on someone, such that they suffer ongoing mental/emotional stress, sleep problems, flashbacks, and/or nightmares. PTSD comes about following physical, sexual, or emotional abuse, neglect, accidents, or even disasters such as war.

A strong connection exists between PTSD and the immune system. PTSD:

- Increases pro-inflammatory cytokines
- Ages the immune system (immunosenescence)
- Causes chronic inflammation
- Can elevate cortisol (the stress hormone) in the long and short term, which impairs immune function
- Can lower cortisol chronically, likely as an adaptive response to chronic stress, increasing the risk of chronic inflammation and autoimmunity
- Reduces the length of telomeres on immune DNA, making it more prone to damage and defects
- Is strongly associated with autoimmune conditions, including rheumatoid arthritis, psoriasis, Crohn's disease, and celiac disease
- Can have a lasting impact on your nervous system by "locking" you into a sympathetic response (the excitatory stress response of the nervous system) or parasympathetic nervous system response (the inhibitory, slowing-down response), which will impair long-term immunity
- Alters genes involved in metabolic processes and immune functioning

Conventional treatment of PTSD is focused on the mind using pharmaceutical and psychological interventions. However, because trauma affects the body, mind, and spirit, any successful intervention must heal all three, not just the mind.

If you suffer from PTSD and a compromised immune system, address the PTSD using a fully integrative approach, and you are likely to see big improvements in immune health too. Consider seeking out a psychotherapist or counselor, along with a bodyworker, healer, shaman, or other mind-body therapist.

TAKE CARE OF YOUR BRAIN'S IMMUNE SYSTEM

Your brain is so important it has its own private immune system and multiple layers of immune protection. Surrounding the brain and spine is cerebrospinal fluid, which houses different types of protective immune cells. Next you have the protective barrier, known as the blood–brain barrier (BBB). And inside of the brain and spine you have microglial cells, which are specialized immune cells that performs multiple roles. They account for 10 percent of all brain cells. These microglial cells perform immune and other roles, including:

- Pruning back dead synapses (nerve cell junctions), which helps you to forget old habits, memories, and learnings, making space for new ones
- Repairing damaged neurons
- Searching the nervous system for foreign invaders or injury in order to destroy any potentially harmful invaders
- Responding to harmful pathogens by fighting them, sounding the alarm so other immune cells can join the attack, and opening the BBB to allow the other immune cells in
- Providing pro-inflammatory and anti-inflammatory effects

They can also potentially damage the brain and spine, leading to disease states such as inflammation, stroke, neurodegenerative diseases (Alzheimer's and depression), and microbial infections.

Similar to the immune system outside of the brain and spine, the microglia are adaptable and have both beneficial and harmful effects. Which effects they offer come down to the conditions presented, which are mainly determined by your lifestyle. Negative stress (distress), pathogenic infections, autoimmune conditions, alcohol, and smoking all trigger the microglia into harmful inflammatory responses. Exercise, improvements in mental health, good sleep, and a healthy diet rich in plant compounds trigger their beneficial responses.

CUT DOWN ON ACID-FORMING FOODS

The digestion of food breaks it down into acid and alkaline bases. The acid-alkaline (pH) balance of your body is extremely important to your health, and in order to maintain this delicate balance, the body uses three mechanisms: the lungs, blood buffering systems, and the kidneys. You influence your blood pH via your diet and breathing.

The body copes with an excessively acidic or alkaline diet for a short period, however a strongly acidic or alkaline diet for a prolonged period causes problems. Especially because, alongside aging, a highly acidic diet degenerates the kidneys, reducing their capacity to regulate pH. An overly acidic state (acidosis) is associated with immune suppression and conditions known to impair immune function (e.g., type 2 diabetes) while an overly alkaline state (alkalosis) has not been found to have any detrimental immune effects.

Most people eat a diet that is excessive in acid-forming foods and low in alkaline-forming foods. Common acid-forming foods include meat, fish, dairy, whole grains, legumes, salt, and soft drinks. Common alkaline-forming foods include fruits, vegetables, and green tea. Neutral foods include most oils and fats, nuts, and seeds. For optimal immune health you need a balance of each group.

You can further explore the pH of food based on its potential renal (kidney) acid load (PRAL) score using an online PRAL chart. To assess the acidic-alkaline balance of your diet, multiply the weight of the food (grams) by their PRAL score.

INVEST IN YOUR HEALTH

The main reason why many people do not invest the time or money in taking good care of their health is simply because they don't value it. It may be uncomfortable to confront, but the excuse that you don't have the time or money to live a healthier lifestyle just isn't true.

For many people, the pursuit of money, material wealth, and career success is a high priority. In the process of pursuing them, they sacrifice sleep and exercise, working excessively and mainly eating convenient, processed foods. True, having lots of money and possessions isn't a bad thing on its own, but sacrificing health in pursuit of them is ill-advised.

The focus on wealth and success is often driven by a belief that money and material objects bring happiness and life satisfaction. Society, the media, and, for some, even friends or family teach this idea. But when you examine the facts of this, it's surprising just how inaccurate it is. Research has explored the relationship between income and emotional well-being. While results vary by country, for most developed countries, $65,000–95,000 USD has been identified as the threshold for a happy and content life. Incomes above this fail to bring any greater happiness or life satisfaction than those within this range. Happiness drops when income is below $65,000 because financial struggles and poverty become commonplace.

This is important to understand because many people are mistakenly sacrificing their immune health, relationships, and personal hobbies, in pursuit of financial/material wealth that will do nothing for their sense of happiness or fulfillment.

How true is this for you? Reexamine what you may be sacrificing in the pursuit of your own goals and make your health a priority.

TAKE VITAMIN C

The most popular vitamin supplement for immune support is vitamin C—and for good reason. Vitamin C improves the production and protection of many types of immune cells, messengers, and antibodies. It is also needed for wound healing and the production of collagen, which is needed for skin and the mucosal lining of the digestive and respiratory tracts (both of which keep harmful pathogens out). When consumed with iron-rich food, vitamin C increases iron absorption—essential for the immune system. Vitamin C reduces the duration and severity of colds, but only protects against colds in those who do high volumes of exercise. Vitamin C is effective at lowering stress, anxiety, and depression, all of which suppress immunity.

Vitamin C is an antioxidant, proven to lower inflammation. Because of its antioxidant properties, some health experts recommend against taking high amounts (500+ milligrams per day) for long periods. This is because too much vitamin C can actually weaken the body's built-in antioxidant system; like any unexercised muscle, it misses out on the challenges (oxidation) needed to grow. Vitamin C can't be stored in the body since it is water soluble, and must therefore be consumed in your diet every day. Foods rich in vitamin C include raspberries, strawberries, blueberries, kiwis, oranges, chili and bell peppers, broccoli, kale, spinach, pomegranate, and lemon.

The recommended daily intake of vitamin C is 75 milligrams for women (120 milligrams for pregnant and breastfeeding women) and 90 milligrams for men. With intakes above 1 gram per day, less than 50 percent is absorbed, and intakes greater than 2 grams may cause digestive complaints. At the onset of illness, take 1–2 grams across the day of liposomal vitamin C (vitamin C in liposomal form doubles its absorption rate).

DRINK MORE WATER

Water plays important roles in virtually every system of the body—and the immune system is no exception. Specifically, the amount of water you are drinking impacts the lymphatic, circulatory, and digestive systems, which all host immune cells.

Dehydration is known to:

- Raise cortisol levels, inhibiting immune function
- Lower levels of SIgA, an important immune antibody found on the mucosa of the lungs and digestive tract
- Trigger inflammation in the lungs
- Thicken the mucus found in the sinuses and respiratory organs, reducing their ability to trap and eliminate pathogens
- Thicken the blood, compromising the transportation of oxygen and immune cells to areas they are most needed
- Thicken the lymph and cause lymph nodes to swell, compromising the lymphatic system's ability to transport immune cells in the body

The best way to keep your body hydrated isn't to drink eight glasses of water a day, however. The most accurate and individualized way is to pay attention to the color of your urine. If you are well-hydrated it will be a pale yellow color. But if it's a dark yellow it's a sure sign of dehydration. If it's consistently clear and free from any color it can indicate overhydration.

Overhydration, though less common than dehydration, can also create health problems, as your bodily fluids become diluted—lowering electrolyte concentration levels, which can lead to weakness, muscular spasms, irregular heart rate, confusion, or nervous system or bone disorders. Hydration isn't just about the amount of water you drink but how you spread that intake across your day. Drinking water in small amounts consistently throughout the day is best, rather than drinking one or more full glasses of water at once.

TAKE CARE OF YOUR SKIN

Your skin is much more than just a container for your body: It's your body's largest organ and part of the immune and detoxification systems. When it comes to your immune health specifically, your skin:

- Forms the barrier that protects you from potentially harmful invaders
- Houses over one thousand different types of microbes: your skin microbiota, which consists of trillions of microbes living within the multiple layers of your skin
- Houses specialized immune cells, messengers, and antibodies that help protect you from outside invaders
- Collects vital information about your environment that supports its development (e.g., exposure to people, nature, and animals brings new microbes and antibodies)
- Is where the body creates vitamin D following sun exposure

Like all other organs, your skin needs nurturing to do its job well. Take care of it by:

- Avoiding chemical toxins used in commercial personal care products and makeup, which can kill or agitate skin microbiota and immune cells
- Going out in nature and enjoying skin contact with the earth, people, and animals to help develop skin immunity and skin microbiota
- Minimizing use of sunscreen, as it blocks most of the UVB light needed to produce vitamin D and contains harmful chemicals
- Filtering your shower/bath water, as chlorinated water dries out the skin and kills beneficial skin microbes
- Avoiding excessive sun exposure, which damages skin

Also be sure to do the basics each day for healthier skin: Eat a healthy diet, drink plenty of water, get plenty of sleep, don't use cigarettes, and avoid or at least reduce alcohol consumption.

SHAKE IT OFF

When you experience stress, especially intense or chronic stress, it doesn't disappear when your circumstances change or when you distract yourself with food, TV, alcohol, etc. It accumulates within your body. To better understand why, it helps to think of stress as a charge. When stressed your nervous system becomes excited; this is why you feel agitated, tense, and unable to relax. The excitement, or charge, needs to be released for the nervous system to return to its normal calm state.

When the negative charge of stress builds up in the nervous system, you may struggle to sleep, your muscles may be chronically tense, your blood pressure and heart rate may be elevated, and you may get ill easily.

Learning to release this stress is important to your well-being and immune health. One powerful way to do this, especially when stress is intense or chronic, is by shaking. It's true: Many mammals shake to release tension especially following trauma or conflict. According to trauma expert Peter Levine, we have this same neurogenic tremor mechanism built into us. A powerful technique for activating this mechanism is Trauma or Tension Release Exercise (TRE). TRE incorporates a sequence of exercises that trigger this tremor response. TRE isn't just good for releasing stress, but also past trauma. You can learn about TRE online, or check out a class in your area.

PAY ATTENTION TO MOON CYCLES

For millennia, many cultures have spoken about the moon's influence on human behavior, psychology, and physiology. The patterns of the moon influence the tides of the ocean and behavior of many animals, birds, and insects. While the moon enters several phases throughout its 29.5-day cycle, the most influential are the full moon (brightest moon) and new moon (darkest moon).

Some studies have indicated changes in sports performance and psychological disorders in connection to the phases of the moon. Research also shows crime, road accidents, and hospital admissions for some conditions increase by up to 5 percent during a full moon.

Although no research has been done into whether lunar phases affect the immune system directly, research has been done into related fields. Many complain of difficulty sleeping during a full moon. Studies show that during a full moon it can take longer to fall asleep, total time asleep is reduced, and lighter phases of sleep are observed. Melatonin levels drop while serotonin levels rise. Melatonin affects sleep and regulates immunity, so when melatonin levels suffer so does immune health. Parasite activity also increases during this time which makes sense as serotonin aids parasite motility. Serotonin increases combined with lowered immunity creates the perfect conditions for parasite activity and may explain the disturbed sleep in some.

Given that the full moon impacts sleep and melatonin levels, it can be worth taking extra precautions during this period, such as using immune and sleep support (e.g., supplementing with melatonin or herbs, foods, or nutrients that help prevent illness such as garlic, colostrum, spirulina, Schisandra, or vitamin D3), especially if you often get ill during this time.

ENJOY RAW HONEY

Raw honey isn't just delicious—it also has immune-boosting properties! It:

- Contains vitamins, minerals, and phytonutrients that boost immunity
- Contains plant compounds that have anti-inflammatory effects
- Helps reduce systemic inflammation seen in inflammatory disease
- Contains phytonutrients that strengthen your antioxidant system
- Is antimicrobial
- Promotes wound healing
- Contains prebiotics that support your gut microbiota
- May have anticancer effects

Avoid buying honey that has been treated above 110°F, as this damages the enzymes found in the honey and may also affect some of its other beneficial nutrients and compounds. Some honey is made from corn syrup to look like honey. This is more likely to occur with cheap honey. Cheap honey is also unlikely to contain the immune-boosting compounds found in the high-grade honey used in studies. Additionally, the farming methods used in the production of low-cost honey means it often contains heavy metals, pesticides, and antibacterial agents, making it more harmful than healthy. Most soft-set honey is raw, so that's a good guide when looking to make a purchase.

There are many different types of honey, each with its unique set of properties and benefits that vary according to flower or bees used in its production, so find one that provides the benefits suited to your needs. Manuka honey, for instance, is a high-quality, medical-grade honey that has been used in traditional and modern medicine for its proven antimicrobial benefits in treating wounds and infections. Adding raw honey to hot foods or beverages damages its beneficial nutrients, compounds, and enzymes, so only add it once they have cooled.

TAKE CHLORELLA DAILY

Chlorella is a freshwater alga that comes from Japan, where it is commonly added to foods like rice and tea. It's packed with nutrients important to immune system function, including various B vitamins, vitamin C, magnesium, iron, zinc, copper, potassium, calcium, chlorophyll, and omega-3. It also contains vitamin B12, which is very rarely found in plants.

Studies examining its effects on the immune system show that chlorella increases natural killer cells and boosts immune antibodies such as SIgA. This makes it particularly beneficial to exercise enthusiasts and athletes prone to colds, as large volumes of exercise often lower SIgA levels.

Studies have also shown that chlorella:

- Provides antioxidant benefits and is particularly effective against advanced glycation end products, a significant source of oxidative stress from food (e.g., sugar or overcooked meat)
- Has anti-inflammatory properties, meaning it lowers inflammatory markers such as c-reactive protein, total cholesterol, and low-density lipoprotein
- Minimizes the inflammatory response involved in allergies and can help reduce lung inflammation (e.g., asthma and COPD)
- Regulates blood sugar levels and improves diabetes
- Aids the detoxification of heavy metals (including lead, cadmium, mercury, and aluminum) and chemical toxins (including dioxin)

Studies typically use dosages between 1.5–10 grams per serving while most chlorella supplements recommend 2–3 grams per serving. It can be consumed as a powder, capsule, or liquid. Chlorella can be added to food, smoothies, and juices or taken as you would any other supplement. It's important to find a good quality, non-toxic source that you trust so that you gain from all its benefits.

BOOST YOUR MELATONIN LEVELS

You may already know that melatonin is an important hormone for sleep, however its biological effects go far beyond this. Melatonin impacts the immune system in many different ways, including:

- Preparing the body for sleep
- Triggering various circadian rhythm processes
- Regulating cellular autophagy (cell recycling) and apoptosis (cell suicide)
- Regulating inflammatory pathways and immune cytokines
- Modulating the immune system (downregulating or upregulating its function as required)
- Regulating immune cells, especially lymphocytes
- Regulating both Th1 and Th2 pathways, which control immune cell response
- Combating oxidative stress in its role as an antioxidant
- Lowering free radicals in the microglial cells of the brain, thereby lowering brain inflammation
- Protecting mitochondria from oxidative damage
- Stimulating the production of glutathione, the other main antioxidant produced by the body

Low levels of melatonin are even linked to autoimmune conditions. You can boost your melatonin levels to aid immunity by:

- Practicing good sleep hygiene
- Avoiding blue light sources at night
- Filtering fluoride from your tap water
- Avoiding fluoridated toothpaste
- Snacking on pistachios, which contain the highest levels of melatonin of all foods

- Using melatonin supplements when needed, such as when experiencing insomnia or jet lag
- Getting plenty of sunlight during the day and darkness at night
- Minimizing use of medical drugs that suppress melatonin (e.g., NSAIDs)
- Boosting daytime serotonin levels
- Avoiding caffeine, nicotine, and tobacco at night
- Minimizing cortisol (the stress hormone), which inhibits melatonin release at night

MIX UP YOUR WORKOUTS

Exercise can provide many benefits that will support immune health. And while all forms of exercise lower inflammation and improve immune health in general, the specific effects vary depending upon the type and intensity used.

Anaerobic exercise is high intensity and usually done for short periods of time—no more than an hour. Many forms of high-intensity exercise exist, though high-intensity interval training (HIIT) and/or strength/resistance training are the most common. HIIT workouts entail repeated bouts of short periods of exercise (a few seconds to a few minutes) performed at a high intensity (>80 percent heart rate max), followed by a short recovering period. This cycle is typically repeated for up to forty-five minutes total. The big advantage of this type of training is that you gain many of the health and fitness benefits of longer workouts doing much shorter workouts. Studies show that short intense forms of HIIT such as Tabata training are the most effective way to improve mitochondrial function, which improves immune health. These workouts are also more effective at strengthening the body's antioxidant system (which reduces oxidative stress and inflammation) than longer workouts.

Resistance training reduces chronic inflammation, which is very damaging to immune function. This occurs because it builds muscle, increases calorie expenditure (metabolic rate), and reduces insulin resistance. A calorie excess and/or insulin resistance causes inflammation.

Aerobic exercise (aka endurance or continuous steady-state exercise) can also improve immune health, although it's important to watch duration with these workouts. The depletion of glycogen stores in the liver and muscles is linked to a drop in immune function. Depending on fitness level this can begin after about sixty minutes of exercise. Moderate-to-high-intensity workouts for longer than ninety minutes can depress immune function for up to three days. For these reasons, from an immune perspective it is better to work out for no longer than sixty minutes if the workout consists of continuous exercise.

Exercise styles originating from the East such as yoga, qigong, and Tai Chi provide unique immune health benefits. They cause much less damage to the tissues of the body (caused by intense/continuous muscle contraction) and emphasize the breath and mindfulness or meditative states. They are particularly effective at lowering stress and strengthening parasympathetic function, which raises immunity and improves states of stress, depression, and anxiety, all known to lower immunity.

Because of the diverse and unique immune benefits of each type of exercise, it is recommended to include as many as possible into your exercise plans. Try mixing things up every other workout session, and remember to take rest days where needed.

ACTIVATE AUTOPHAGY

Autophagy is the process by which cells degrade and recycle their dysfunctional parts. *Auto* means "self," while *phagy* means "to eat," so autophagy essentially means to eat oneself. Luckily, it's far more beneficial than it sounds! Autophagy is highly beneficial to immune health because it:

- Optimizes cell function including that of immune cells by allowing the body to replace faulty cell parts or cells completely
- Replaces dysfunctional mitochondria (mitophagy) that may be producing excessive levels of oxidative stress
- Prevents the buildup of toxins created by infections
- Removes harmful microbes from inside cells (xenophagy)
- Modulates the immune response to infections
- Reduces inflammation in the long term
- Inhibits the growth of early onset cancers
- Inhibits pro-cancer processes such as DNA damage and chronic inflammation

You can trigger or enhance autophagy by:

- Fasting
- Restricting calories
- Doing aerobic exercise
- Eating a ketogenic (low-carb) diet
- Moderating your coffee consumption
- Sleeping (this is optimized when combined with not eating 3–4 hours before bed)

You can also consume any of the following to trigger or boost autophagy:

- EGCG (polyphenol found in green tea—best taken for immune health as an extract or via matcha green tea)
- Resveratrol (polyphenol found in grapes—best taken for immune health as a supplement)
- Curcumin
- Vitamin D
- Nicotinamide
- Omega-3

There are lots of ways to activate autophagy. Try out the options that work best for your lifestyle.

TAKE ELEUTHERO

Eleuthero, also known as Siberian ginseng, is an East Asian adaptogenic herb. It was traditionally used to increase energy and decrease stress, but more recently has been enjoyed for its immune benefits. Siberian ginseng is the distant cousin of American and Asian ginseng, though it has very different effects.

Eleuthero's important compounds include:

1. **Eleutherosides:** Fight cancer and improve diabetes
2. **Oleanolic acid:** An antioxidant
3. **Ursolic acid:** Anti-inflammatory, fights cancer and improves diabetes

Eleuthero increases immune cells (T lymphocytes and natural killer cells) and antibody response (IgG and IgM). Some research suggests that it's effective against RNA viruses (e.g., colds and flu) but not DNA viruses (e.g., herpes). When used to fight colds and flu it needs to be taken as soon as symptoms appear for the full benefit.

Eleuthero is an effective anti-inflammatory that works by blocking the inflammatory enzyme (COX-2) and improving lymphatic system function. Its anti-inflammatory effects likely arise from its antioxidant properties.

Other effects of eleuthero include:

- Inhibiting mast cell activity, making it effective at reducing allergy symptoms
- Building resilience to stress and strengthening stress recovery, reducing risks of illness
- Regulating blood sugar levels by increasing insulin sensitivity, improving diabetes and immune function

Eleuthero comes in a number of forms, including tincture, solid extract, powder, tea, capsule, and tablet. Dosage varies by condition so be sure to look into what amount is best for you. For the common cold, 400 milligrams 1–3 times a day is often recommended; in dried form 2–3 grams per day is recommended. Be sure to buy eleuthero only from a reputable and trusted source. It can interact with medications, so check with your doctor before using eleuthero. Eleuthero has immune-stimulating and anti-inflammatory effects, so approach with caution if you suffer from autoimmunity.

USE THE RIGHT HERBS

If you have an allergy or autoimmune condition some herbs can make your condition worse while others can improve it.

One of the main immune cells released in response to an invader are T helper cells. These cells can be divided into two main types—T helper 1 (Th1) and T helper 2 (Th2) cells. (Other pathways exist, but these are the main two.) Th1 cells are activated when an intracellular immune response is required and are mainly pro-inflammatory and linked to most autoimmune conditions. Th2 cells are activated when an extracellular immune response is required and are mainly anti-inflammatory and increase allergy reactions.

Th1 and Th2 pathways work like a seesaw so only one is dominant at a given time. A healthy immune system is balanced between the two and switches between each when required. However, when one always dominates, problems arise.

It's important to know which pathway is dominant in your condition, as some herbs trigger a Th1 response (e.g., *Panax ginseng*, echinacea, and astragalus) while others trigger a Th2 response (e.g., turmeric, green tea, and resveratrol). If you are Th1 dominant and you take a Th1 herb it will make your condition worse. However, if you take a Th2 herb it can create balance, improving your immune health and condition.

You can find the dominance of your condition online, as well as which side a given herb stimulates. The most accurate way of determining your Th1:Th2 dominance, however, is to run a test with your doctor using a Th1:Th2 cytokine blood panel, as dominance can vary in some conditions.

If you have an allergy or autoimmune condition use only herbs that support the weaker side of the seesaw.

EXPLORE MEDICAL ASTROLOGY

Astrology is an ancient science, practiced across almost every culture throughout time. The Mayans, Egyptians, Greeks, Chinese, Arabs, Indians, and Western Europeans all practiced astrology and—despite being in separate parts of the world—came to surprisingly similar conclusions.

Astrology is the study of how the celestial bodies of our solar system influence our psyche, personality, physiology, and life events. Everything centers around your birth (natal) chart: a map of where each of the planets were relative to earth when you were born. You can find a free copy of your natal chart online.

Medical astrology is a branch of astrology focused on health and physiology that was practiced by Western doctors until the seventeenth century. It tells you which organs and systems are likely to be impaired and what ailments you are likely to suffer. By understanding this you can take more focused preventative steps to safeguard your health.

In medical astrology, the zodiac signs (twelve signs that reflect the position of the sun when you were born), planets, and houses (twelve positions that align with Earth's twenty-four-hour rotation around its axis) correspond to specific areas of the body, systems, and ailments. The sun and moon have the greatest influence, although certain planets are more relevant to immune health. Planets that have the greatest immune influence include Neptune (immune/lymphatic system), Mars (inflammation), and Pluto (infections). However, because many organs/systems influence immunity, this doesn't rule out the influence of the other planets. The first house of your chart reflects your capacity for health, while the sixth, eighth, and twelfth houses correspond to pathology and disease.

If you're new to astrology, consider seeking the help of someone experienced in medical astrology to interpret your chart.

UNDERSTAND THE MENSTRUAL CYCLE

The hormonal fluctuations that take place during the menstrual cycle influence the immune system, effectively making the female immune system cyclical. This has important implications to infection risk and immune-related conditions (allergies and autoimmune disease). The menstrual cycle has distinct phases:

1. **Follicular phase.** This phase sees elevations in estrogen, immune antibodies, and inflammation. This helps prevent pregnancy and strengthens the body in preparation for pregnancy. Allergies and autoimmune symptoms are likely to flare up during this phase.
2. **Early-mid luteal phase.** This phase sees elevations in progesterone and drops in estrogen. During this period, the immune and inflammatory responses are suppressed due to ovulation. This maximizes the chance of pregnancy by preventing the immune system from attacking the egg or sperm. During this phase infection risk is greater and autoimmune/allergy symptoms are likely milder.
3. **Late luteal and menstruation phases.** During these last two phases both progesterone and estrogen are low and the inflammatory response returns, so inflammatory conditions may worsen.

Hormone-based birth control uses synthetic forms of estrogen or progesterone intended to thicken the womb and prevent ovulation. Synthetic estrogen pills may increase inflammation but lower infection risk, while progesterone pills can reduce inflammation and increase infection risk.

Lifestyle factors such as sugar, inflammatory foods, poor sleep, and stress can all elevate estrogen and suppress progesterone levels, while heavy metals (e.g., cadmium and nickel) and chemical toxins (e.g., xenoestrogens) can mimic the effects of estrogen in the body. Stress also increases inflammation and risks of autoimmunity. Living a healthy life-style and minimizing stress positively affects these hormones.

If you get ill frequently, particularly during the early luteal phase of your menstrual cycle, consider using immune support during this phase by supplementing with vitamin C, echinacea, and/or vitamin D3. If your autoimmune conditions flare up during the follicular or late luteal phase use anti-inflammatory support such as supplementing with an omega-3, eleuthero (Siberian ginseng), Ashwagandha, or *Panax* (Asian) *ginseng.*

PAY ATTENTION TO THE SUN

Did you know that activity of the sun one hundred million miles away affects the way your nervous and immune systems work?

That may seem a little far-fetched but there is a good deal of evidence and science to back it up. Activity on the sun is not constant and happens in cycles. These solar cycles are marked by periods of low sunspot activity (solar minimum) and periods of high sunspot activity (solar maximum), which alternate between the two every 5–6 years, with one complete cycle lasting 10.5–11 years. According to NASA the end of sunspot 24 and beginning of sunspot 25 is the year 2020, and 2019–2021 is the lowest period of sunspot activity in over two hundred years. The next high sunspot activity begins around 2025.

When a sunspot appears on the sun, solar flares are emitted and take at least eight minutes to reach the earth. Fortunately, the earth's ionosphere protects us from this radiation—otherwise we would all be fried by now. Nonetheless this electromagnetism still affects life on the earth.

Researchers have observed a strong pattern between high or low sunspot activity and human activity. Solar maximum is linked to periods of high excitability which are experienced as either intense global conflict and tension (such as international conflict, wars, riots, crime, and revolutions) or extraordinary levels of innovation and creativity (such as in the arts, sciences, social change, and financial markets). Solar minimum is linked to times of low energy and activity on the planet, where repression and pandemics are usually seen. The 2020 COVID-19 pandemic is a good example of this.

While high and low levels of sunspot activity are linked to mass human effects, it is not limited to this. Solar radiation also affects personal human health and activity. Strong solar radiation emitted from solar flares and solar wind causes strong geomagnetic storms which are believed to affect the nervous system and the pineal gland (produces melatonin to regulates sleep and the immune system) in the human brain, both of which are sensitive to electromagnetism. This can disrupt circadian rhythms (sleep) and melatonin release, which play important roles in immune health. Geomagnetic storms are also linked to elevations in depression, suicide, and cardiovascular-related incidences. Solar flares can cause you to feel anxious, jittery, dizzy, irritable, lethargic, and exhausted. Either can affect you for days—not just during the elevated period.

These solar changes do not predict events, of course, but they do provide us with the framework or theme of what to expect. They can also provide advance warning of when to take precautions, avoid high-risk situations, and do more to lower stress and support our immune and nervous systems. Understanding this activity can also help you to better understand why you feel the way you do, aiding peace of mind and immunity. You can learn more about current and forecasted solar weather patterns at www.swpc.noaa.gov.

DRINK COCONUT WATER

Coconut water is touted as nature's sports drink due to its high levels of electrolytes (essential minerals), which is of a similar electrolyte balance to your blood. Coconut water comes from young coconuts, also called green coconuts, which have not fully matured. As they mature, the nutrient-dense water found in the coconut is used to produce the white meat of the coconut.

Coconut water is a particularly good source of magnesium, manganese, and potassium but also contains levels of the immune-boosting nutrients calcium, sodium, and vitamin C. Because of its electrolyte content it is effective for hydration.

Several studies have shown coconut water to be effective at reducing inflammation and lowering inflammatory cytokines and other inflammatory markers. Although water from mature coconuts has some anti-inflammatory effects, water from young coconuts is significantly more effective at lowering inflammation. It has also been shown to activate antioxidant responses, regulate blood sugar levels and cholesterol levels, and improve conditions such as diabetes and cardiovascular disease.

The best source of coconut water is from fresh green coconuts. Once opened, the water should be drunk within 3–5 days. Avoid coconut water products that have been pasteurized (much of the nutrients are lost in this process) or those made from concentrate or made with sweeteners or flavorings. If you are buying packaged coconut water you want one that has been produced using cold pressure and contains nothing but coconut water, preferably organic.

GO ORGANIC

Eating organic food is a simple change that you can make in order to support your immune system. Consuming organic rather than commercially farmed foods is better because food grown in accordance with organic farming principles has been proven to contain higher levels of vitamins, minerals, antioxidants, and phytonutrients that are needed to support a healthy immune system. Organic foods are also farmed using much lower quantities of agricultural chemicals (e.g., pesticides, herbicides, insecticides, etc.), antibiotics, and growth hormones. Ideally organic foods are completely free of these farming chemicals and hormones, but this varies between organic certifications—some types are allowed.

The reason organic plants and animal products contain higher levels of nutrients and lower levels of chemicals is because organic farming methods are different from commercial farming methods. The soils in organic farming methods are much healthier and more nutritious, meaning the plants are also healthier and more nutritious. Animals are reared according to much higher welfare standards and fed healthier diets, so they are also healthier and do not require the same levels of antibiotics and vaccines in order to survive. They are usually grown at natural rates as well so growth hormones are not usually used.

The one exception is organic fish. To be certified organic it must be farmed, and farmed fish (organic or otherwise) are highly stressed and parasite-ridden, unlike their wild counterparts.

Familiarize yourself with the main organic certifications of your country and the standards and practices required to meet them. Then look out for those symbols on the labeling of the products that you buy. Always go for organic foods that meet the highest farming standards set out by the organic certification body.

Of course, organic foods tend to be a lot pricier than non-organic foods. If organic foods are out of your budget:

- Use the Environmental Working Group's (EWG) lists of the Dirty Dozen and Clean Fifteen to guide your choices: These are the fruits and vegetables grown with the highest/lowest levels of pesticides
- Buy non-organic produce that is grown without pesticides and animal produce from grass-fed, hormone-free, and/or free-range animals
- Soak fruits and vegetables in apple cider vinegar or sodium bicarbonate before consuming them to remove the agricultural chemicals found on their exterior
- Grow your own fruits and vegetables without using chemicals

TAKE A LUNCHTIME WALK

A simple yet powerful way to improve your well-being *and* immune health in one hit is to go for a walk at lunchtime. This has many immune-boosting effects, including:

1. **Stress reduction.** Taking yourself out of the office helps you take a mental break from any sources of work tension.
2. **Movement.** Moving throughout the day is vital to strong immunity.
3. **Sunlight.** Exposing your skin to sunlight at lunchtime boosts vitamin D levels and exposes your skin to blue, red, and infrared light—all proven to enhance your immune system.
4. **Deeper breathing.** Taking a few deep conscious breaths while going for a short walk reduces stress, gets you back in the present moment, and allows your immune system to function better.
5. **Nature.** Try to take your walk in nature or a local park, as it provides many immune-boosting benefits and reduces stress.
6. **Connection.** Socializing helps release stress and improves immune health in a host of ways. Share your walk—and its benefits—with a friend or colleague!
7. **Blood sugar regulation.** Going for a light walk after eating increases insulin sensitivity and regulates blood sugar levels, which strengthen immunity.
8. **Balanced circadian rhythm.** Regular daily movement develops a strong, balanced circadian rhythm and aids sleep, both essential to immune health.

In one study, researchers found that walking for twenty minutes a day five times a week reduced the number of sick days participants took by 43 percent. In multiple studies it has been shown that 30–45 minutes of brisk walking five times a week protects against respiratory infections.

WATCH OUT FOR THE BIG EIGHT

The "big eight" are eight foods your immune system is most likely to react to. This reaction is known as a food allergy or food sensitivity. A food sensitivity is sometimes called an intolerance, hidden food allergy, or non-IgE food allergy. An allergy is a strong (sometimes life-threatening), almost immediate immune reaction. A food sensitivity is a much milder immune reaction that involves less aggressive immune cells and antibodies and can take hours or days to appear.

The eight most common foods that trigger immune reactions are:

1. Milk
2. Eggs
3. Fish
4. Crustacean shellfish
5. Tree nuts
6. Peanuts
7. Wheat
8. Soy

If you react to any of these foods it will trigger an inflammatory response and may include discomfort or even pain. These reactions compromise your immune system for a couple of reasons:

- They can damage the gut lining, allowing harmful pathogens to enter the body
- As long as your immune system is busy attacking the foods you are eating, it has less capacity to defend you against harmful invaders

If you react to any of these foods you should eliminate them from your diet. If you suspect an allergy or sensitivity to a food, you can try eliminating the food for 2–3 weeks, then reintroducing it by consuming lots of it for twenty-four hours. This will provoke a strong reaction if your immune system reacts to the food.

APPLY THE PEACE AND HARMONY APPROACH TO YOUR IMMUNE SYSTEM

The immune system is often discussed as a system of defense and attack. And it's therefore often believed that a healthy immune system is always on edge, seeking out invaders so it can mount an attack. But as Matt Richtel pointed out in *An Elegant Defense: The Extraordinary New Science of the Immune System*, the true nature of the immune system is not focused on attack and defend, but on peace and harmony. This may still mean attacking when that's appropriate but it can also mean withdrawing or doing nothing.

This is an important distinction to make, because your understanding of the nature of your immune system determines the actions you take to improve it. If you view the immune system as a system of attack and defense, it's no wonder you will seek out ways in which to strengthen and boost immune system function. However, this approach can have harmful consequences. Seeking to stimulate and armor up the immune system via pharmaceutical or more natural solutions comes with the risk of developing an immune system that becomes oversensitive or overactive. Autoimmunity can arise and both allergies and autoimmunity are made much worse when the immune response is excessively active.

This same view of the immune system has also led society to numb the immune system when it is found to be overactive. Immunosuppressive drugs used in autoimmunity are an example of this. The limitation of such approaches is that they leave users with a handicapped immune system incapable of responding effectively to pathogens or cancer. Consequently, many suffering autoimmune conditions eventually develop many other debilitating and harmful conditions. These solutions have their place, of course, but they are not an effective long-term solution.

Instead of trying to strengthen the immune system for an attack, the goal should be to educate and integrate your immune system into the world as much as possible. Get out into nature and enjoy plenty of contact with other people as well as plants and animals. In doing so you empower your immune system to work intelligently with the rest of your body *and* the world around it. Taking this approach will enable the immune system to better self-regulate and respond to threats at an appropriate level. This is how you build a healthy, optimally functional immune system that prevents you from getting unnecessarily ill—with minimal risk of developing immune complications.

PRACTICE INTERMITTENT HYPOXIC BREATHING

A hypoxic state refers to a state of reduced oxygen availability in the cell(s). Intermittent Hypoxic Breathing (IHB) is a type of breathing that creates this state. IHB is simply a means of reducing cell oxygen levels for a short period of time on an intermittent interval basis.

You may wonder why you would want *less* oxygen. Temporary states of hypoxia bring about many health and immune benefits, including:

- Lowered inflammation
- Increased levels of cell mitochondria (more mitochondria means stronger immune system)
- Enhanced initial immune response without increased inflammation
- Improvements in insulin resistance, cholesterol levels, obesity, type 2 diabetes, and metabolic syndrome
- Improved depression
- Increased immune cell numbers
- Alterations to over five thousand genes, including genes important to your immunity

There are different IHB techniques out there, the most famous being the Wim Hof Method. You can learn more about this method online. Another simple but effective and convenient method is walking IHB:

1. While walking and after exhaling your breath fully, hold your breath for as long as you can (be gentle the first few times you do it).
2. After releasing the breath-hold through the mouth or nose, return to normal breathing (ideally through the nose).
3. Once you have recovered, repeat the first two steps 4–12 times.
4. Count your steps or measure time and distance when you hold your breath and try to increase these amounts over time.

WASH YOUR HANDS WISELY

Washing your hands is an easy hygiene practice that helps prevent infection. It has been shown to:

- Reduce illness with diarrhea by 23–40 percent
- Reduce diarrheal illness in those with weakened immune systems by 58 percent
- Reduce respiratory illnesses, like colds, by 16–21 percent
- Reduce sick days in schoolchildren due to gastrointestinal illness by 29–57 percent

However, there is a downside to this practice. The health and development of our immune system, especially as children, requires exposure to microbes. So being overly hygienic such as washing your hands too often can actually weaken your immunity.

There is a fine balance to be had: You want to expose your body to plenty of microbes to keep your immune system fit, while at the same time avoiding the pathogenic ones that create illness. For this reason, washing your hands after using the bathroom, before eating, before handling food, and after handling raw meats/seafood is a must. However, there is much debate about washing hands at other times. There may be a good argument for washing hands after using public transport, especially because many pathogenic germs can be passed on that way and the average person touches their face sixteen times an hour (including vulnerable areas like the nose and eyes where infections are easily transmitted).

When washing your hands, lather them with soap then wash for at least twenty seconds in all areas, including between fingers and underneath nails. Wash your hands at important times but don't overdo it.

GO RED

Of the different types of light, the current consensus within the scientific community is that the most beneficial are red and infrared light wavelengths.

Both red and infrared light are found in nature via sunlight and fire, which we were once exposed to day and night. In contrast, modern lifestyles are spent indoors almost the entire day and rarely in front of a fire. Both red and infrared have similar effects; only the depth they penetrate varies, with near-infrared penetrating the deepest, impacting different tissues. Infrared heat also brings some unique benefits as well.

Red and infrared benefit your immune system by:

- Reducing inflammation
- Improving autoimmune and chronic inflammatory conditions
- Strengthening the body's internal antioxidant system
- Increasing energy (ATP) production by the cells' mitochondria
- Increasing oxygenation of the cells
- Promoting wound healing
- Stimulating the lymphatic system (transports immune cells around the body and eliminates toxins and waste products)
- Stimulating the production of stem cells, which can potentially become active immune cells
- Increasing melatonin production, which regulates both sleep and immune function
- Improving mood and emotional state (including anxiety and depression, which lower immunity)
- Improving skin tissue (an important immune organ)

The simplest way to increase your exposure to red and infrared light is to get out into sunlight. Finnish saunas and infrared saunas are another great way to boost infrared light exposure. Another option is to purchase a specialized red and infrared light therapy device.

EAT AN ANTI-INFLAMMATORY DIET

It's clear that the two biggest threats to your immune health are chronic stress and chronic inflammation, with stress itself being a major inflammatory. Luckily, there are many ways to reduce both threats, and diet plays a major role.

You can reduce sources of inflammation in your diet by cutting out or at least reducing the following inflammatory foods:

- Sugar-rich beverages (sugar-sweetened drinks and fruit juices)
- Sugar-rich foods (cookies, candy, cake, ice cream, chocolate)
- Refined carbohydrates (white bread, white pasta, white rice)
- Processed meats (hot dogs, ham, bacon, sausages, smoked meat)
- Processed snack foods (crackers, chips, pretzels)
- Inflammatory oils (processed nut, seed, and vegetable oils)
- Hydrogenated oils (processed foods containing hydrogenated ingredients)
- Alcoholic beverages

You should also aim to eat no more than three ounces of meat per day and reduce red meat intake to three or less servings a week. Avoid commercially farmed meats that are high in (inflammatory) omega-6s. Avoid cooking meat and other foods at high temperatures, especially when grilling or frying meat.

You can also counteract inflammation by enjoying foods rich in compounds and nutrients that have anti-inflammatory effects, including:

- Cruciferous vegetables (broccoli, kale, Brussels sprouts, bok choy, cabbage, cauliflower, spinach)
- Berries (strawberries, raspberries, blueberries, blackberries, grapes, cherries)
- Fat-rich plants (avocados, coconut, olives)

- Healthy fats (olive oil, coconut oil)
- Fatty fish (salmon, sardines, herring, mackerel)
- Nuts (almonds, walnuts, pecans)
- Peppers (bell peppers, chili peppers)
- Cacao (dark chocolate, raw cacao powder)
- Herbs and spices (turmeric, ginger, fenugreek, cinnamon)
- Tea (green tea)

An anti-inflammatory diet doesn't have to feel restrictive. Incorporate these great alternatives and additions into your meals.

HEAL YOUR GUT

The mucosal lining of your gut is a critical part of your immune defenses. Part of its job is to prevent unwanted invaders from getting into the body. Food and microbes don't technically enter the body until they pass through this barrier, which runs through the respiratory tract and from the mouth to the anus as one giant tube. In the intestines, this tube is just one cell thick so that food and water particles can be absorbed effectively. The problem with having such a thin protective layer is that if anything goes wrong with it, you are in trouble. This is why 80 percent of your immune system and gut microbes are located there, so that they can protect it. However, there are many factors that can reduce immunity and harm the gut microbiota and epithelial cells of the intestines, including:

- Processed foods
- Chlorinated water
- Alcohol
- Nonsteroidal anti-inflammatory drugs
- Chemical toxins
- Electromagnetic stress
- Emotional stress
- Pathogenic infections (harmful bacteria, fungi, parasites, etc.)
- Antibiotics
- Late-night eating
- Insomnia
- Gluten (for some)

Many of us encounter these triggers through choice or circumstance on a regular basis. When this happens, in high doses or over a prolonged period of time, the gut's immune system (namely the antibody SIgA) becomes suppressed, the microbiota is damaged, and the intestinal lining becomes damaged, inflamed, and permeable (also known as "leaky gut"). And when this happens, the tight junctions between intestinal cells that keep everything out open up and unwanted food particles, chemical toxins, and harmful microbes can enter the body, causing illness and compromising well-being. As these unwanted invaders enter the body, the immune system identifies them as the enemy and begins attacking them. This causes the symptoms associated with food sensitivities/intolerances. In some cases, especially with a hypersensitive/overactive immune system, the immune system can confuse these unidentified invaders with the tissues of the body, potentially leading to an autoimmune condition. Many health experts believe that intestinal permeability plays an important role in the development of autoimmune conditions.

Unfortunately, you can't heal a leaky gut overnight or by simply taking a few magic pills for a few weeks. It is a process that can take weeks, sometimes months, and involves eliminating all causes of harm to the gut, avoiding foods you may have developed sensitivities toward, healing any harmful microbial infections, detoxifying the body, and providing the nutrients and herbs required to heal the gut.

Fortunately you can take a more proactive approach to protect your gut by minimizing your exposure to many of these causes of gut permeability and by supporting a healthy gut microbiota. If you suspect that the lining of your gut is damaged, seek the help of a professional trained in functional medicine, nutrition, or naturopathic medicine.

USE ASHWAGANDHA TO BOOST IMMUNITY

Ashwagandha, also called "Indian ginseng," is an adaptogenic herb from India that is commonly used in Ayurvedic medicine to reduce stress. As an adaptogenic herb, it helps your body to react or recover from short- or long-term stress. Ashwagandha has many effects on the body—many of which benefit the immune system, including:

- Increasing immune cells including macrophages, natural killer cells, and other lymphocytes
- Increasing immune antibodies
- Offering antimicrobial, antifungal, antiparasitic, and antiviral effects
- Reducing inflammation
- Lowering pro-inflammatory cytokines
- Reducing inflammatory markers including c-reactive proteins, triglycerides, and total and low-density lipoproteins
- Lowering stress, anxiety, and depression
- Lowering cortisol (the stress hormone) levels
- Increasing insulin sensitivity
- Improving blood sugar regulation
- Improving diabetes
- Offering antioxidant properties
- Improving quality of sleep and decreasing the time it takes to fall asleep
- Potentially killing cancer cells

Ashwagandha extracts can be taken as a supplement in various forms including powder, capsule, pill, or essential oil. Studies have used 120–1,200 milligrams per day. The dosage typically recommended for capsules is 300–500 milligrams, taken once or twice a day.

CUT OUT INFLAMMATORY FATS

One important aspect of your diet is the quality of fats you consume. Many commonly used fats and oils can damage your health and provoke harmful inflammatory immune responses, leading to chronic inflammation and impaired immune health.

You can cut inflammatory oils from your diet by:

- Avoiding any foods that contain hydrogenated oils
- Removing all types of extracted polyunsaturated oils (e.g., vegetable, nut, seed, or fish oils) and consuming omega-3 and omega-6 fatty acids only from whole foods
- Consuming monounsaturated oils (but do not cook with them and be sure to store them in cool, dark cupboards or the fridge!)
- Only cooking with saturated oils and fats

Fats and oils are delicate and easily damaged by heat, light, or oxygen making them inflammatory. As soon as you extract an oil from a plant or animal source you are directly exposing it to heat, light, and/or oxygen. In fact, some extraction processes even generate heat.

Oils contain different balances of three types of fatty acid that determine their vulnerability. Some contain mainly polyunsaturated fatty acids (omega-3 or -6) such as nut, seed, vegetable, or grain oils. Others contain predominantly monounsaturated fatty acids (omega-9) such as olive or avocado oil. And some contain predominantly saturated fatty acids such as butter, ghee, or coconut or palm oils. Polyunsaturated oils are very easily damaged by the elements, making them the most unsafe to consume in extracted form. Additionally, oils rich in omega-6 (e.g., sunflower, safflower, corn, soybean, and vegetable oil) trigger inflammatory immune responses regardless of whether they have been damaged. In their undamaged state, omega-3 fatty acids trigger anti-inflammatory responses; however, once damaged, they develop inflammatory properties. In general, oils rich in monounsaturated fatty acids are safe to consume in extracted form as long as they are high-grade, sealed in dark bottles, and cold-pressed. Fats and oils rich in saturated fatty acids are the least easily damaged by the elements and are safe to consume in extracted form.

Saturated fats are often portrayed as harmful to human health, but this is not accurate. Excessive amounts of foods rich in saturated fat can be unhealthy, but the same argument can be made for any type of fat consumed in excess. You can enjoy saturated fats in moderate amounts alongside a balanced intake of the other fatty acids.

The final most inflammatory of oils/fats are hydrogenated oils, also called trans or cis fats. These are unsaturated oils that have had hydrogen added to them through a manufacturing process called hydrogenation in order to make them more solid. These fats should be avoided completely. They are sometimes used in processed foods and should be labeled on the food packaging.

REDUCE OXIDATIVE STRESS

Oxidative stress occurs as a result of an excessive buildup of reactive oxygen species (ROS), a type of free radical. A free radical is an atom or molecule with one or more unpaired electrons, making it highly reactive or "radical." When the body is unable to balance these ROS with neutralizing enzymes or antioxidant compounds, cells or tissue are damaged by oxidative stress. Chronic and excessive levels of oxidative stress cause chronic inflammation, damage to DNA and proteins, and eventually degenerative or autoimmune diseases. Chronic inflammation and autoimmunity disrupt healthy immune function.

Oxidative stress at controlled levels is perfectly healthy (e.g., exercise), and some immune system responses even produce oxidative stress. The body regulates ROS and oxidative stress by producing neutralizing enzymes and antioxidants, supported by external sources of antioxidants.

Unhealthy levels of oxidative stress are the result of:

- A weak internal antioxidant system (the main mechanism for neutralizing ROS)
- A lack of antioxidants from external sources
- Excessive quantities of ROS (mainly caused by lifestyle)

You can support your body to combat excessive oxidative stress by:

Strengthening your internal antioxidant system through:

- Regular exercise
- Eating lots of plant foods (high in phytonutrients that strengthen the internal antioxidant system)
- Exposure to sunlight
- Improved sleep (melatonin is your body's main antioxidant)
- Hypoxic breath-holding

- Avoiding antioxidant supplements (they weaken this system)
- Regular sauna use
- Cold thermogenesis (e.g., cold showers)
- Fasting

Increasing antioxidants from external sources by:

- Eating lots of antioxidant-rich foods (plants)
- Grounding to the earth (barefoot contact with the earth)

Minimizing your exposure to external man-made sources of ROS, which include:

- Inflammatory foods
- Processed foods
- Refined sugar
- Cigarettes
- Alcohol
- Chemical toxins
- Pollution
- Heavy metals
- Electromagnetic stress
- Emotional stress
- Pesticides
- Some medications

Minimizing oxidative stress in your daily life will go a long way in improving your immune health.

TURN TO A TRUSTED FRIEND

Friends play many roles in our lives—including influencing our immune health! Aside from the joy of friendship, and the social and physical contact that friends bring (which are proven to benefit immunity), friends can also offer important emotional qualities that influence immunity, such as empathy.

During times of emotional stress, we are most vulnerable to infection. Empathy, which is defined as the ability to understand and feel the emotion of another from their perspective, provides strong benefits to the immune system. One study found that patients with cold or flu symptoms saw a 50 percent improvement in immune response (SIgA) when the doctor they visited displayed strong empathy in contrast to those who didn't. In a similar study, researchers found that doctor empathy was linked to significant reductions in inflammation, as well as duration and severity of colds. Empathy unquestionably improves the capacity to heal.

Receiving empathy isn't limited to just friends or family, although they are your most reliable source. Plan ahead and make sure you have someone close by to talk to, who truly understands you and won't spend that time advising or telling you what to do. This could be your spouse, family member, work colleague, or friend. Ensure that they are able to listen and display the empathy you may need during difficult times—and make sure you can be that empathetic person for someone too. Research shows that demonstrating care and compassion for another improves your own immune health.

USE THESE OILS TO SUPPORT YOUR IMMUNITY

Essential oil use is a branch of botanical medicine that provides many different health benefits including immune benefits. The oils extracted are produced by the plant to protect itself from harmful microorganisms. Like other plant extracts the oils contain potent beneficial properties.

Essential oils can affect your immunity in many ways from stimulating or suppressing the immune system to providing anti-inflammatory, antioxidant, antiseptic, or antimicrobial effects. Common essential oils and their benefits include:

1. **Bitter orange.** Antioxidant, anti-inflammatory, and antifungal, and combats anxiety.
2. **Clove bud.** Antimicrobial and antiseptic and fights viral infections.
3. **Cinnamon.** Cleans surfaces and the air.
4. **Eucalyptus.** Antiviral, antibacterial, anti-inflammatory, and antioxidant; stimulates the immune system; and helps fight respiratory infections.
5. **Frankincense.** Anti-inflammatory, antioxidant, and antimicrobial, and stimulates the immune system.
6. **Lavender.** Reduces stress, aids sleep, reduces depression, and provides anti-inflammatory and antioxidant effects.
7. **Lemon.** Antioxidant and antibacterial, and aids immune function (especially in the respiratory system).
8. **Niaouli.** Fights parasites and viral infections.
9. **Oregano.** Anti-inflammatory, antibacterial, antiviral, and antioxidant, and helps fight infection.
10. **Palmarosa.** Antibacterial, antifungal, and antiviral, and stimulates the immune system.

11. **Peppermint.** Antibacterial and antifungal and protects against colds and the flu.
12. **Rosemary.** Antibacterial, helps fight respiratory infections, and cleans the air.
13. **Tea tree.** Stimulates the immune system and is antimicrobial.
14. **Thyme.** Antibacterial, stimulates the immune system, and combats respiratory infections and coughs.

When using essential oils, always dilute the oil into water or a carrier oil such as coconut, castor, or avocado oil, as undiluted oils can irritate the skin, eyes, nose, throat, and lungs. Essential oils should never be consumed orally unless specifically designed for it. Purchase only organic, pure forms, and store in glass bottles. Essential oils can be used via a diffuser, bath, massage, steam inhalation, or hot/cold compress.

RESOLVE IRON DEFICIENCY

Iron is required for healthy immune function and low levels are damaging to your health and immune system. Specifically, iron is needed by the immune system:

- For the production and healthy function of many kinds of immune cells
- For the production of immune messengers (cytokines)
- To prevent the degeneration of the thymus gland, an important immune gland
- To produce red blood cells that provide the oxygen that enables the immune system to function

Recommended iron intake is 8 milligrams per day for adults. (For menstruating women, it is 18 milligrams per day.) If you are vegetarian or vegan it is a good idea to exceed this amount, since plant-based iron is less easily absorbed.

You can increase your iron intake by:

- Eating foods rich in iron and/or taking an iron supplement
- Consuming vitamin C (e.g., orange juice) with iron-rich foods to enhance iron absorption
- Identifying and resolving any underlying non-dietary causes behind iron deficiency with the help of a health professional

Foods rich in iron include animal organs (offal), meat, fish, poultry, nuts, seeds, and leafy greens. These sources are not equally balanced though, as plant-based iron is less easily absorbed by the gut. Why? It comes down to two reasons: First, because plants contain phytates and oxalates, which block the absorption of iron and other minerals; and second, because nonheme (plant) iron is not as easily absorbed as heme (blood/animal) iron. Soaking or sprouting grains, nuts, and seeds overnight is recommended to help break down phytates. However, phytates provide health benefits, so it's best not to do this all of the time. Cooking grains and leafy greens also breaks down oxalates and phytates, however, cooking also reduces levels of some micronutrients, so it's good to eat both raw and cooked greens. A healthy balanced gut microbiota is also important, as some strains of bacteria break down oxalates.

Iron deficiency in the body isn't always caused by a lack of iron in the diet. It can also be caused by excessive levels of copper or zinc, inflammatory conditions (e.g., autoimmunity), digestive problems, heavy menstruation, or pathogenic microbial infections (some microbes steal iron from cells as it is needed for their growth).

If you choose to use an iron supplement to boost iron levels, always consume it with food and ideally use iron gluconate, as it has the highest absorption rate. Don't take an iron supplement based upon the assumption that you are iron deficient; get your iron levels checked first via a blood test by your doctor or other health professional, as iron overload (usually seen with intakes of 45+ milligrams per day) is harmful.

CARE FOR A PET

Compared to our ancestors we have a vastly different relationship with microorganisms. The mass introduction of antibiotics along with better hygiene brought about by sanitation, garbage collection, pasteurization, cleaning products, and city living have greatly reduced our exposure to microbes. Research has revealed that this is a double-edged sword: While it has allowed us to thrive on the planet, our reduced exposure to microorganisms has damaged the development of our immune systems. The "Old Friends" hypothesis developed by scientists explains that the surge in autoimmune conditions and allergies over recent decades is directly linked to this drop in exposure, especially at a young age when our immune system is developing.

Your exposure to microorganisms teaches your immune system how to regulate itself. Without frequent and diverse exposure there is a greater risk of it becoming hypersensitive (causing allergies) or less capable of distinguishing self from non-self (causing autoimmunity).

Pets expose you to many types of microbes you wouldn't otherwise come into contact with, which aids your immune development. This is especially important for children growing up in city environments where exposure to animals and nature are limited.

Research shows that a lack of exposure to nature and animals is also detrimental to mental health, further weakening immunity. One study found that depression levels are higher in adults who grow up in city environments without a pet. Pets also improve mood, lower stress, and encourage you to be more active (dogs especially), all of which improve immunity.

BEFRIEND HEALTHY ROLE MODELS

Famous motivational speaker Jim Rohn once said that you are the average of the five people you spend the most time with. And research backs this up. Social psychologist Dr. David McClelland found that the people you habitually associate with determines 95 percent of your success or failure in life. Analysis of an ongoing seventy-year health study of thousands uncovered that if your friend became obese, you were 57 percent more likely to gain weight. If a friend of your friend became obese, you were 20 percent more likely to gain weight—even if you didn't know them personally. And if a friend of the friend of your friend developed obesity, you had a 10 percent greater chance of gaining weight. Similar risk patterns were also seen with smoking.

Those around you clearly have a huge influence over your choices and outcomes. This is true across all areas of life; your immune health is no different.

The habits, thought patterns, and emotional well-being of those within your social and familial circles rub off on you. This can be both good and bad news. If you want to upgrade your lifestyle and immunity, the fastest and easiest way is to spend less time with those who indulge in the habits you wish to change and spend more time with those who have already adopted your desired habits.

Make change easier by finding and spending more time with role models who have the lifestyle and health you want for yourself.

PRACTICE PRANAYAMA

Pranayama is a practice of breath control used in yoga through a variety of different techniques before and after yoga postures.

As with other breathing techniques, pranayama can bring a whole host of physiological effects known to benefit immune health. These include reductions in stress, anxiety, depression, and cortisol (the stress hormone); stimulation of the parasympathetic nervous system (calms down the nervous system and supports immune health, digestion, and detoxification) and lymphatic system (transports immune cells and eliminates toxins and waste products); improved blood acid-alkaline balance; and improvements in sleep. Pranayama has even been found to affect 25 percent (that's five thousand!) of the genes in your body.

In terms of direct immune effects, it lowers inflammation and increases immune cells (neutrophils). One study found that twenty minutes of pranayama reduces inflammatory markers, while other studies have found that it effectively reduces lung inflammation, improving asthma and chronic obstructive pulmonary disease (COPD). Asthmatics benefit most from breathing exercises in pranayama that emphasize the outward breath.

There are many different pranayama techniques, but those most beneficial to immunity are:

1. **The Humming Bee Breath (Bhramari).** Good for stress, anxiety, anger, melatonin, and sleep.
2. **Forehead Shining Breathing Technique (Kapalbhati).** Best for boosting that immune system, but also good for stress, intestinal problems, diabetes, constipation, asthma, allergies, and sinusitis.
3. **Alternate Nostril Breathing Technique (Anuloma Viloma).** Helps with stress, bronchitis, asthma, diabetes, arthritis, and acidity.
4. **Breath of Fire (Bhastrika).** Good for digestion; the spleen, pancreas, kidneys, liver, stomach, intestines, nervous system,

sinuses and tonsils, colds, flu, sinus, asthma, throat problems, allergies, stress, and anxiety.

5. **Chanting Breath Technique (Udgeeth).** Good for insomnia, the nervous system and digestive system, acidity, anxiety, tension, stress, and anger.

Learn more about these techniques online, and experiment to find those that work best for you. Begin by practicing a few minutes a day and increase practice over time.

TRY SOUND HEALING

Sound technology is a powerful way of affecting your physical, mental, and emotional health. Research by Dr. Mitchell Gaynor, former director of medical oncology at Cornell's Center for Integrative Medicine, helped bring to the world the science behind the healing power of ancient sound technologies like chanting and Tibetan and crystal singing bowls. Specifically, he found that like ultrasound, certain sound frequencies can kill cancer cells and activate specific immune cells and messengers.

Other studies have shown that sound technology affects mental processes, muscles, the nervous system, heartbeat, pulse, and digestive and circulatory systems and creates an overall relaxed feeling.

Sound healing technology such as Tibetan and crystal singing bowls, gongs, mantras, and chanting create a deeply relaxing meditative state that:

- Releases emotional stress such as anxiety
- Lowers cortisol (the stress hormone)
- Releases endorphins (feel-good hormones)
- Lowers brainwave patterns (from stress states to calm and stillness)
- Stimulates the immune system
- Reduces inflammation and fibromyalgia

Sound healing works through entrainment and resonance that influences cells to vibrate at the same frequency as the sound. A helpful analogy is the vibration of a tuning fork, which, when struck, can activate another tuning fork of the same frequency (tone) simply through soundwaves. By creating resonance within the tissues and cells of the body, sound healing moves cells from a state of incoherence (stress), where cells vibrate at different frequencies, toward coherence (health), where they vibrate at the same frequency. This is the natural healthy state in which immune and other cells and systems function best.

GET OUT AND GARDEN

Gardening is one of the most effective ways to boost your immune system—it's true! Here are eight reasons why:

1. **Exercise.** Gardening will get you moving and exercising your body in ways you otherwise wouldn't.

2. **Sunlight and fresh air.** Gardening gets you outdoors and benefiting from the immune-enhancing effects of sunlight and fresh air.

3. **Microorganisms.** One gram of soil contains up to ten billion microorganisms. The "Old Friends" theory explains that losing your connection with microorganisms through modern hygienic living weakens your immunity. Getting your hands dirty is critical to re-establishing a healthy connection with microorganisms.

4. **Better mental health.** Gardening lowers anxiety, stress, and depression—which lower immunity—and has been used successfully in horticultural therapy for treating mental health.

5. **Nutritious foods.** Growing your own food allows you to lower your intake of pesticides (which harm immunity), increase nutrients in your diet, and try your hand at growing immune-boosting foods.

6. **A connection to nature.** Gardening provides you with the immune benefits of grounding (connecting with the earth via your bare skin, usually barefoot) and phytoncide (oil with antimicrobial properties that is released by trees and plants).

7. **Human connection.** Gardening is an opportunity to connect and foster deeper relationships with friends and family, which strengthens immunity.

8. **Healthier diet.** Growing your own food deepens your connection with and appreciation for real food and leads to healthier dietary choices, especially among children.

EXPERIMENT WITH PEMFS

Conventional medicine and the health sciences view the body as a physical and chemical system, however newer and emerging sciences view it as electromagnetic. And the electromagnetic nature of the body plays vital roles in how your cells and biochemistry function. In fact, some health experts believe it governs biochemistry. They argue that degenerative health conditions begin with electromagnetic disruptions that lead to biological disruptions. Through these newer ideas, the use of electromagnetic therapies such as PEMF, or pulsed electromagnetic field, are becoming more popular.

PEMFs are low-level electromagnetic fields that operate at similar frequencies to those found in nature. Unlike man-made EMFs, which are harmful and cycle up to several billion times more than those found in nature, PEMF technology uses much lower frequencies, between 1 and 10,000 Hz. In fact, most treatments use under 30 Hz, lower than the frequency experienced in a typical thunderstorm.

Studies have found that PEMF therapy:

- Strengthens all cell types
- Helps regulate the immune system
- Lowers inflammation and inflammatory cytokines and markers
- Combats autoimmune conditions and allergies including rheumatoid arthritis, fibromyalgia, and asthma
- Helps the body fight bacteria and viruses
- Improves depression
- Improves blood sugar regulation
- Promotes wound healing
- Improves sleep
- Reduces cell hypoxia

Learn more about PEMF therapy online and talk to your doctor to determine whether it's a good fit for you.

TAKE AN INTEGRATED APPROACH

There are tons of different variables at play when it comes to shaping your immune health. All of these factors, lifestyle *and* environmental, interact with one another and can weaken your physiological, psychological, and emotional systems. Poor choices in one area (e.g., an unhealthy diet) make you susceptible to the harmful effects of others. For example, if you eat a diet lacking in plant foods that help build the body's antioxidant system, you will be much more vulnerable to the harmful effects of free radicals produced by electromagnetic fields. Your environment is especially impactful, as modern technologies and practices have led to an abundance of harmful elements, including toxic chemicals, heavy metals, and electromagnetic fields.

If you want to see serious improvements in your immune health, you need to take an integrated approach, rather than working to heal just one area of your life. Examine each part of your lifestyle and environment: What might be causing you harm? What unhealthy decisions in one area might be feeding into negative effects in another? You can use the following as a guide, or as a jumping-off point for your examination:

- Lifestyle factors (physical): diet, exercise, gut health, vaccinations, medications, sleep, breath, hydration
- Lifestyle factors (mental): emotions, social connection, attitudes, mental health
- Lifestyle factors (spiritual): spiritual connection, beliefs, energetic blocks, nature connection
- Environmental factors: chemical toxins, heavy metals, electromagnetism, light exposure, time spent in nature

You are a holistic being made up of many systems—tangible and intangible, personal and social—each one affecting the other. Make changes slowly but make them holistically, addressing your environment, mind, and body.

EAT LESS MEAT

There is much debate about the health benefits and harmful effects of meat, especially red meat, and the answer is certainly not clear-cut. When it comes to immune health, most of the harmful effects are inflammatory-related:

- Meat increases inflammatory markers such as c-reactive protein
- A sugar found in animal meat is known to trigger inflammatory responses, since the immune system doesn't recognize it and sees it as a threat
- High levels of advanced glycation end products, which cause oxidative stress and inflammation, are found in processed or over-cooked meat (which typically occurs when it's grilled or fried)
- Red and processed meats can cause oxidative stress, inflammation, and cancer
- Meat is rich in the amino acid L-carnitine, which has inflammatory effects
- Meat contains amino acids that trigger insulin release and contribute to insulin resistance, a known cause of inflammation and diabetes
- Commercially farmed animals are fed high-grain diets, making their meat rich in omega-6 oils, which are inflammatory
- Commercially farmed meats contain traces of antibiotics, growth hormones, and other agricultural chemicals that interfere with the body's biochemistry, microbiota, and immune system

Cutting out meat can significantly reduce inflammation, especially if you normally eat a lot of it. However, this is not always the healthiest course of action. Vegetarians and vegans typically have lower levels of immune cells and antibodies and they often lack nutrients important to immune health, including omega-3 oils, vitamin D, vitamin B12, zinc, iron, and other minerals. This is because many plant sources of these nutrients are not absorbed as easily, or the form these nutrients are found in is not as efficiently converted into a usable form within the body. Some studies also show that non-meat eaters are more prone to colds, flu, and allergies.

On the upside, vegetarians typically have much lower levels of inflammation—in part due to a meatless diet, but also because many plant foods are rich in antioxidant and anti-inflammatory compounds.

To improve your immune health while ensuring your body gets the nutrients it needs:

- Consume meat only from free-range, grass-fed animals (preferably from organic or wild sources)
- Avoid processed meats
- Avoid browning or cooking meat at high temperatures (e.g., grilling or frying)
- Restrict meat intake (not including seafood) to no more than 2–3 ounces (50–80 grams) per day
- Consume a diet rich in whole plant foods (particularly fruits and vegetables), which help mitigate the inflammatory effects of meat

TAKE 100 PERCENT RESPONSIBILITY

For many, it's easier to blame poor immune health on everyone and everything but themselves. After all, who likes admitting when they've made a poor decision? The reality is that your current state of health is the direct result of your lifestyle, environmental, personal, career, familial, and social choices. The only way to change your health is to take responsibility for these choices and make intentional changes moving forward. No *ifs*, *buts*, or excuses—choose and act.

Strong immune health begins with personal responsibility. Rather than relying on outside forces to tell you what is or isn't good for you, take ownership and research it yourself. And if you are skeptical about anything you read, that's good: A healthy dose of skepticism keeps you safe. Investigate and ask questions. Try not to dismiss anything just because it sounds a little unusual, extreme, inconvenient, or not "you," either. Your health today is the result of who you've been and what you've done up until this moment. Resisting change keeps you stuck. Choose to be 100 percent responsible for your lifestyle and health education and build from there.

TRY CBD OIL

Cannabidiol (CBD) oil is one of over one hundred cannabinoid compounds found in the cannabis plant. Unlike marijuana, it doesn't contain the psychoactive compound tetrahydrocannabinol (THC), responsible for the "high" when smoking or taking an edible.

CBD oil has been found to have stimulating and/or suppressive effects on the immune system. In autoimmune conditions CBD oil can suppress inflammatory responses by inhibiting the CB2 receptor in the brain, which is the part of the endocannabinoid system that controls immune/inflammatory responses. Additionally, it suppresses pro-inflammatory cytokines and the reuptake of adenosine (an anti-inflammatory) in the brain. While immunosuppressive drugs shut down the entire immune response, increasing risks of infection and cancer, CBD oil appears to suppress only inflammatory immune responses. CBD oil may also support those with weakened immunity. Studies in cancer patients found that it increased natural killer cells and cancer cell apoptosis (cell suicide).

Other immune-related benefits of CBD oil include improvements in:

- Anxiety and depression
- Sleep and insomnia
- Inflammation
- Numerous inflammatory, allergy, and autoimmune conditions
- Type 2 diabetes

CBD oil can react with some medications, so seek professional guidance before adding it to your health regime. Talk to your doctor/health specialist before using CBD oil if you're immune impaired, as much is still unknown.

CBD oil can be taken via capsules, tinctures, epidermal creams, oils, or transdermal patches. Ensure the oil is certified for its purity. Many factors influence dosage so do your own research to determine what amount is best.

ADDRESS NON-PHYSICAL CAUSES OF IMMUNE IMPAIRMENT

Immune impairment arises for many reasons. And while most people relate to the physical causes of impairment, the non-physical causes can be just as important—even more so—and may be at the root of the problem.

A common non-physical cause of impairment is emotions. Emotional and psychological problems don't just stem from the mind; often they are the result of emotions and/or trauma that get trapped in the body when you don't fully process or experience your emotions. For example, you may shut down or distract or numb yourself because the experience and emotions tied to it are too overwhelming. These emotions can then accumulate and affect you on a deeper level, leading to tendencies toward distressing emotional states such as anxiety, anger, or depression. And when you are in a distressed state much of the time, your immune system can become chronically suppressed as a result. If you experience emotional challenges, getting professional help from a trained therapist, somatic bodyworker, or other mind-body therapist can be valuable—not only for your immune health, but your happiness and well-being too.

There are also other ways to work with the blockages and imbalances created within the body. Your body has energy channels and centers in which energy (your "life force") flows. These are what are known as chakras and energy meridians. Sometimes blockages in these cause immune problems and other physical, emotional, or psychological problems. To unblock and rebalance your own energetic body, visit a practitioner trained to work with these subtle energies, such as an energy healer, Reiki practitioner, shaman, bioenergy medicine practitioner, tantric masseuse, Traditional Chinese medicine practitioner, medical qigong therapist, acupuncturist, or other similar therapist.

TAKE SPIRULINA

Spirulina is an alga that grows in some lakes of West Africa and Mexico. It provides many different health benefits, including those for your immune system. It has direct effects on immune cells including macrophages, natural killer cells and other lymphocytes, and immune antibodies. Some research also suggests that the compounds it contains may even help protect immune cells from stress and damage. Spirulina has strong antioxidant effects and helps to strengthen the body's own antioxidant system. It also lowers levels of pro-inflammatory cytokines and prevents histamine release. (Its histamine effects may partly explain why studies have found that it benefits hay fever.) What's more, it lowers inflammatory markers, including total cholesterol and low-density lipoproteins (LDLs), and may protect LDLs from free radical damage. It also regulates blood sugar levels and protects against diabetes.

New research also suggests that it may help to prevent viral infections. Spirulina contains immune-supporting nutrients, including vitamins B1, B2, B3 and E as well as iron, copper, and other minerals such as magnesium. It also contains another immune-boosting nutrient, polysaccharides, which stimulate spleen, thymus, and bone marrow activity.

So how do you reap all these great immune benefits? When it comes to supplementing spirulina, you can take it in pill, capsule, or powder form. Most studies have used servings of 2–10 grams per day. No harmful effects are known, so it is safe to take amounts on the upper end of this range. Natives to the lakes where it originates consume it in much higher quantities. Because of its effects in boosting immune function, it is not advised to use spirulina if you have an autoimmune condition, especially lupus, multiple sclerosis, or rheumatoid arthritis.

MITIGATE THE HARMFUL EFFECTS OF WI-FI AND CELL PHONES

Of the three main types of electromagnetic fields (EMFs), research shows that by far the most harmful are radio frequency (RF). Wi-Fi and cell phones are your main sources of radio frequency fields.

The immune-related effects of these high-frequency EMFs include:

- Overstimulated or suppressed immune cell responses
- Strong links to numerous allergy (mast cell responses) and auto-immune conditions
- Damage to the blood–brain barrier, which can lead to neurological/ neuropsychological effects (including depression and early-onset Alzheimer's) and means the brain and nervous system are vulnerable to damage from chemical toxins, heavy metals, harmful microbes, and the nervous system's own specialized immune system
- Damage to the lining of the gut, which increases infection risk
- Damage to cell membranes, meaning cells have less control over what goes in or out of the cell, possibly increasing the risk of intra-cellular viral and bacterial infections
- Interference with cell calcium channels, which leads to high levels of cell damage, oxidative stress, and inflammation
- Damage to cell mitochondria, which diminishes ATP production (without ATP cells, the immune system cannot function)
- Inflammatory responses in the skin
- Suppressed melatonin production, which disrupts sleep and immune regulation
- Links to blood sugar dysregulation and diabetes
- Links to numerous cancers and childhood leukemia
- Damaged cell DNA and irreversible genetic mutations

- Damage to the gut microbiome balance
- Attacks on bacteria, which can lead to the development of antibiotic-resistant bacteria strains

Not all of these effects will happen to everyone all of the time, as many variables influence the effects of high-frequency EMFs, including intensity, duration, frequency of exposure, the area most frequently exposed (e.g., head, groin, etc.), genetics, biological weaknesses, and health status. These effects apply to children tenfold, as their bodily tissues (especially vital organs) are much more vulnerable to the effects of EMFs while their bodies are still developing.

You can help mitigate some of the harmful effects of Wi-Fi and cell phones by:

- Not carrying your cell phone in your pocket
- Turning your cell phone on flight mode when not in use, especially when carrying it on your person
- Turning your cell phone off or onto flight mode at night
- Using a protective cell phone case proven to reduce EMF exposure
- Using an air tube headset or speakerphone when speaking on your phone (wired and Bluetooth headsets are harmful)
- Using wired internet at home, or at least turning off your Wi-Fi at night
- Avoiding putting laptops and mobile devices on your lap

NURTURE YOUR SPIRITUAL LIFE

Spirituality and immune health are more connected than you may think! In fact, a comprehensive review by researcher Harold Koenig of hundreds of studies examining the relationship between religion and spirituality and physical and mental health confirms this bond. Out of fourteen studies, 71 percent demonstrated a positive association between spirituality/religion and good immune health. In another ten studies, 70 percent found that spirituality/religion was associated with lower viral infection rates. And on examining lifestyle practices, Koenig discovered that spirituality/religion was associated with lower use of alcohol, drugs, and cigarettes; healthier diets; and more exercise. He also showed that religion/spirituality was associated with stronger mental health (lower stress, depression, and anxiety).

Other research shows that those following a spiritual or religious path cope better with stress, experience greater peace and calmness, socialize more, and have greater satisfaction in life—all proven to bolster immune function.

Other benefits of spirituality that boost immunity include:

- Greater meaning and purpose in life
- Frequent experiences of love
- Greater self-esteem and self-worth
- Greater inner peace and joy
- Stronger desires to contribute
- A deeper sense of gratitude
- Deeper bonds with friends and family
- A stronger sense of community

Spirituality is distinct from religion and can take many different forms. It may include practices such as meditation, mindfulness, prayer, yoga, Tai Chi, or qigong. You may choose to attend worship services or other communal events or keep your spiritual activities private. Spirituality might include being in nature or being at home. There is no one "right" way about it.

USE N-ACETYL CYSTEINE

N-acetyl cysteine (NAC) is the supplementary form of the amino acid L-cysteine. L-cysteine is used by the body to produce glutathione, the most abundant antioxidant in the body. Glutathione is poorly absorbed by the body, which is why supplementing it isn't normally recommended. However, NAC supplementation is recommended, as studies show it corrects glutathione deficiency.

NAC's immune-related benefits largely come from its antioxidant effects, which include:

- Counteracting harmful oxidative effects of chemical toxins, radiation, heavy metals, and pesticides
- Removing heavy metals from the body
- Improving recovery from the common cold (viruses cause oxidative stress)
- Reducing inflammatory cytokines and inflammatory markers
- Reducing inflammation and protecting against disease in the lungs (e.g., COPD and infection)
- Reducing insulin resistance (partly caused by oxidative stress)
- Mitigating the chronic inflammation caused by obesity
- Reducing gut inflammation, acid reflux, and leaky gut
- Reducing and protecting against small intestine bacterial overgrowth

NAC also protects against and improves the immune response (natural killer cells) to the flu—particularly in the immunosuppressed such as those with HIV—and aids recovery from the flu. It breaks down the biofilm that bacteria produce to cling to surfaces and protect themselves from attack. This then opens the door for the immune system and antibacterial compounds to kill the bacteria.

Additionally, NAC regulates brain glutamate levels. Excessive levels are linked to psychological disorders and addiction, which lower immunity. NAC's combined glutamate and antioxidant effects also make it perfect for reducing brain inflammation.

Dosages of 1,800–2,400 milligrams of NAC are commonly used in studies, taken across 2–3 servings. For general health, 600 milligrams per day is typically used.

MAINTAIN HEALTHY VITAMIN E LEVELS

There are eight different types of vitamin E, with alpha-tocopherol being the most commonly used in supplementation. The main role of vitamin E is as an antioxidant that protects your cells from oxidative stress. This is particularly important for immune cells, which rely on vitamin E's protection from free radicals in order to do their job. For this reason, vitamin E deficiency can mean big problems for your immune health.

Studies have found that vitamin E supplementation:

- Reduces bacterial and viral infection
- Slows down the progression of HIV/AIDS
- Reduces the incidence of colds and flu in the elderly
- Protects against and improves lung inflammation including asthma
- Reduces cancer risk

Vitamin E deficiency can be caused by smoking, obesity, inadequate intake, genetic mutations, and poor fat absorption in the gut (vitamin E is a fat-soluble vitamin).

The following foods are good sources of vitamin E: sunflower seeds, nuts (almonds, peanuts, and hazelnuts), spinach (and other green leafy vegetables), broccoli, eggs, and kiwi. Wheat germ oil is probably the richest source of vitamin E, however, because it is an extracted polyunsaturated oil and therefore vulnerable to oxidation, its safe use is questionable. Vitamin C and glutathione can both help to keep vitamin E levels up as well, while high-fat meals aid its absorption.

The recommended intake for vitamin E is 15 milligrams daily (19 milligrams for pregnant women). Use caution, as intake above 1,000 milligrams (achieved via supplementation) can cause harmful effects.

PLAY A SPORT

Sports may not typically be considered for their immune-boosting effects, but there are several great reasons to make them a part of your immune defenses:

1. **Exercise.** Exercise is proven to strengthen your immunity, and sports are a fun way to get moving.

2. **Nature.** Many sports are played outdoors, and that means you are breathing fresh air, getting some sunlight, and coming in contact with the earth—all of which boost immunity.

3. **Connection.** Sports get you socializing and connecting with others, especially team sports. Mingling with others, often in close proximity, provides many immune benefits. And if it is a contact sport, that further enhances your immune system, as physical contact means the exchange of antibodies and microorganisms from one person to another, further enhancing immune system function.

4. **Mindfulness.** Most sports require your complete attention. You can't hit the ball across the court while thinking about that project you need to finish at work next week. The nature of sport brings your attention into the present moment and away from stressful thought patterns, reducing stress and enhancing immune function.

5. **Fun.** Sports are an enjoyable pastime. These lighter states of emotion help to release stress and keep the nervous system and emotions in a positive state supportive of the immune system.

Start experimenting to find a sport (or more than one) that you enjoy and try to make it a regular part of your week. There may be club sports you can join in your area. You can also start your own unofficial "team" with friends and set a time each week to meet up and play for fun.

GET PLENTY OF VITAMIN A

Vitamin A refers to a group of fat-soluble compounds that support your health. There are two main types of vitamin A:

1. **Preformed vitamin A (retinoids).** This is vitamin A in its active form that the body can use immediately; it comes from animal sources. Preformed vitamin A includes forms such as retinol, retinal, and retinoic acid.

2. **Provitamin A.** These are carotenes (an important pigment for photosynthesis) and are an inactive form of vitamin A, meaning that to be used they need to be converted into an active form by the body. Provitamin A comes from plant sources and includes alpha-carotene, beta-carotene, and beta-cryptoxanthin.

Vitamin A in retinoic acid form is most important to the immune system. It regulates genes involved in immune function and is needed for the production of white blood cells, especially the different kinds of lymphocyte cells. It is especially important for the production and distribution of T lymphocytes. A lack of retinoids increases your risk of infection, slows down your recovery, and reduces the immune response to immunization.

Retinoic acid also plays a vital role in regulating the health of all mucosal linings within the gut (critical to immune health). It is particularly important in the development of health and function of antibodies in the gut (immunoglobulins). A deficiency of retinoic acid is linked to the development of an intolerant immune system, which means you are at greater risk of developing food sensitivities. A deficiency can also elevate pro-inflammatory cytokines and increase risk of developing autoimmune conditions.

The precursors to vitamin A, the carotenes, have antioxidant properties, which is important for optimal immune function. Because of their antioxidant effects, carotenes provide a protective role against some forms of cancer, while the retinoids inhibit cancer cell growth. Carotenes can also protect against metabolic conditions such as diabetes and metabolic syndrome, which lower immunity.

Both plant and animal sources of vitamin A are important to a healthy immune system. Plant sources include sweet potatoes, pumpkin, butternut squash, carrots, kale, spinach, cabbage, swiss chard, red peppers, and collard greens. Animal sources include egg yolks, liver, butter, salmon, cheddar cheese, mackerel, and trout. Carotenes from plants can be converted to the retinoids but conversion is poor (28:1 ratio), so those eating a vegan diet need to make sure they are consuming plenty of carotenes.

To avoid vitamin A deficiencies, men are recommended to get 900 micrograms and women 700 micrograms (1,300 micrograms for pregnant women) of retinoid vitamin A every day, which equates to about 6,000–15,000 micrograms of carotenes. It's important not to exceed the upper limit of 3,000 micrograms of retinoids, as it is a fat-soluble vitamin, which means it is stored in the body and can be toxic in high amounts.

TONE UP YOUR VAGUS NERVE

The vagus nerve is responsible for your parasympathetic nervous system, which regulates the immune response. It also influences many other areas of your biology and informs the brain of what's going on in most of your organs. For the healthy function of the digestive, detoxification, and immune systems, the vagus nerve must be active much of the time.

Aside from being active, the vagus nerve also needs to be strong and toned. A strong vagal tone means that the body recovers quickly from stress and regulates things like blood sugar and inflammation better. Low/weak vagal tone can lead to chronic inflammation and a weaker regulation of the inflammatory response and immune systems.

You can tone up your vagus nerve through:

- Cold exposure (cold showers or ice baths)
- Singing or chanting
- Gargling
- Yoga
- Tai Chi
- Prayer
- Meditation
- Deep, slow breathing, emphasizing the outward breath
- Socializing
- Exercising regularly
- Laughing often
- Pulsed electromagnetic field therapy

You can measure the strength and responsiveness of your vagus nerve by using a heart rate variability (HRV) app. Some HRV apps (such as SweetBeat HRV) will tell you both how active your vagus nerve is (HRV score) and how toned it is. Track your vagal tone regularly.

MAINTAIN HEALTHY COPPER LEVELS

Copper is a mineral you might not hear much about when it comes to the body, however like all nutrients, it plays important roles in your health. A deficiency or excess of copper can compromise your immunity.

A copper deficiency affects immune cells. It lowers neutrophil activity and numbers and disrupts macrophage activity (macrophages use copper to intoxicate microbes). Both types of immune cells are critical to the initial immune response, so when copper levels are low it increases your risk of infection. Deficiencies in copper also lower T lymphocyte growth and levels of cytokine IL-2. IL-2 regulates the immune system and prevents autoimmune conditions, while T lymphocytes kill infected cells, activate other immune cells, produce cytokines, and regulate the immune response.

A copper deficiency can stem from:

- A lack of copper-rich foods in the diet
- Poor gut health that affects the absorption of minerals including zinc
- Excessive use of antacids
- An excessive consumption of zinc from supplements

As an antioxidant, copper neutralizes free radical damage but at the same time, in excess, can promote free radical damage and inflammation. Copper is also anti-inflammatory, which is why it lowers inflammatory markers, including total cholesterol and low-density lipoprotein, and elevates high-density lipoprotein. Keeping copper in a healthy range is therefore critical to managing both antioxidant and inflammation levels.

Copper-rich foods include liver, shellfish, nuts, seeds, cacao/cocoa (dark chocolate), beans, potatoes, peas, leafy greens, mushrooms, avocados, and dried fruit. The recommended intake of copper is 0.9 milligram per day for adults (1.1–1.3 milligrams for pregnant women). Above 10 milligrams per day causes copper toxicity. If you are using a zinc supplement ensure you are also meeting your copper needs.

SLOW DOWN

While you might think of stress as the result of life circumstances, this isn't the main source of stress. In Western society, the most pervasive source of stress is actually the fast pace of modern life. That constant pressure to go go go makes everything feel urgent, so you have no choice *but* to feel anxious about getting everything done as fast as possible. And since stress suppresses the immune system, one of the simplest things you can do to improve it is to slow down. Stop chasing; stop racing to the top; stop accumulating more—more money, more things, more experiences, more knowledge, etc. Our never-ending pursuit of more wears down our health, creates chronic stress, and impairs the immune system.

The best teacher here is nature. It is never in a rush, never lacking, never trying to get anywhere, yet it is the most productive and consistent force on the planet. Through nature's slowness, much gets done.

Nature operates in seasons. There is a time to begin anew (spring), a time for action (summer), a time to harvest (autumn), and a time to rest (winter). The pace of nature varies by these seasons. If nature operated as we do, it would spend eleven months a year in summer and one week in winter. This may work temporarily, but eventually it would burn its resources. Soils would become depleted, rivers would dry up, animal and plant life would become riddled with disease, and life on the planet would end.

Nature teaches us that if we want to go far and enjoy sustainable results, we must understand that by slowing down we speed up. Life has a natural rhythm and cycle to it: Match that rhythm and you cultivate not only better health, but overall satisfaction.

SPROUT YOUR FOODS

Sprouting is a simple process that can make foods extra beneficial to your immune health. It involves soaking seeds or legumes for several hours then rinsing them a few times a day until they sprout "tails." Sprouting:

- Increases the content of some nutrients including protein, fats, vitamins, minerals, and antioxidants
- Increases enzyme content, which may improve digestion of the food
- Breaks down phytates, lectins, and other antinutrients found in grains and legumes that can limit the absorption of minerals
- Increases the fiber content, which feeds gut microbiota
- Neutralizes acid-forming foods, which suppress immune function
- Improves inflammatory and metabolic conditions

Consuming 60 grams of sprouts every day has been found to improve diabetes. Studies have also found they lower blood sugar levels, total cholesterol, and low-density lipoprotein ("bad" cholesterol) and raise high-density lipoprotein ("good" cholesterol) levels—all linked to better immune health. Some sprouts such as alfalfa are also rich in plant polyphenols (compounds that boost antioxidant and anti-inflammatory responses) and have been proven to lower several inflammatory cytokines.

You can sprout different types of nuts, seeds, beans, grains, and vegetables and use them in tons of delicious recipes, including soups, omelets, rice, salads, stir-fries, and more. Although sprouting is relatively simple it's worth researching to better understand the safest and most effective methods, as they can vary depending on the grain, seed, or legume used. Although most sprouts are eaten raw, some legumes and grains must be cooked after sprouting, as they can be harmful when eaten raw (e.g., kidney beans).

HACK 171

BOOST GLUTATHIONE LEVELS

Glutathione is considered the master (or mother) antioxidant of the body. It's a critical part of your defense against oxidative stress, inflammation, and immune impairment. Unlike most other antioxidants, which come from food, it's produced by the body and recycles other antioxidants, extending their lifespans.

Upon reaching adulthood your ability to produce glutathione diminishes. Once in your forties, deficiency symptoms, such as fatigue, poor sleep, aches/pains, and low immunity, begin to appear. Luckily, there are simple improvements you can make to elevate or maintain glutathione levels, including consuming:

1. **A protein-rich diet:** (Animal products, legumes, nuts, and seeds.) Glutathione is made from the three amino acids found in protein: cysteine, glutamate, and glycine.
2. **Sulfur-rich foods:** (Meat, eggs, fish, grains, garlic, onion, and cruciferous vegetables.) Sulfur contains cysteine and methionine, which are used to make glutathione.
3. **Dairy:** Casein, found in dairy, raises glutathione levels.
4. **Whey protein:** It contains high levels of cysteine.
5. **Selenium-rich foods:** (Meat, fish, cottage cheese, Brazil nuts, and brown rice.) Selenium is needed for glutathione activity.
6. **Glutathione-rich foods:** (Spinach, avocados, asparagus, and okra.) Although dietary glutathione is poorly absorbed, it may provide some benefit.
7. **Turmeric (curcumin):** Curcumin raises glutathione levels—take as a concentrated supplement for significant effect.
8. **Raw liver:** It's a concentrated source of many nutrients and compounds, including glutathione and its supportive nutrients. Only

228

consume liver from organic, grass-fed animals; liver from commercially farmed animals is toxic.

Exercise also boosts your glutathione levels.

Minimize factors that cause oxidative stress and deplete glutathione, including:

- Excessive UV light
- Excessive alcohol consumption
- Smoking
- Sleep deprivation
- Chemical toxins

PROTECT AGAINST VIRUSES WITH ASIAN GINSENG

Originally used to beat fatigue, ginseng has since proven to have a number of immune benefits, particularly against viruses. There are three main types of ginseng: American ginseng (*Panax quinquefolius*), Asian (red or white) ginseng (*Panax ginseng*), and Siberian ginseng (eleuthero).

Compared to American ginseng, there is significantly more research supporting Asian ginseng's use in combating upper respiratory infections (e.g., colds and flu) and, to a lesser extent, other types of viruses and bacteria.

Ginseng gets most of its benefits from five compounds:

1. **Saponins:** Anticancer, lower blood cholesterol and sugar levels
2. **Polysaccharides:** Fight fatigue and lower stress
3. **Ginsenosides:** Anti-inflammatory and antioxidant effects
4. **Gintonins:** Anti-inflammatory and antioxidant effects
5. **Polyacetylene:** Antibacterial

Ginseng raises most types of immune cells and has a favorable effect on immune cytokines. It also increases longevity in those with HIV (an immunosuppressed condition). When used alongside various vaccines (e.g., the flu vaccine) it often boosts their antibody response. Studies have also found that it enhances immunity when recovering from cancer.

Asian ginseng benefits inflammatory lung conditions (asthma and COPD) and respiratory allergies (hay fever). Studies also show it lowers blood sugar levels, suppresses appetite, and aids weight loss, making it of great benefit to diabetics.

The natural root form is thought to be most effective. Typical dosage is 0.5–2 milligrams per day. Dosages as high as 15 milligrams produce unpleasant side effects, so use caution. It should not be used by children or pregnant women. Individuals with autoimmunity should seek professional advice before consuming ginseng of any variety.

TAKE A NAP

The designated nap times of childhood may be in the past, but a regular nap still offers rejuvenating brain and body benefits! On top of helping you feel more alert, napping improves cognitive performance, memory, learning, stamina, emotional well-being, and immune health.

One study found that sleep deprivation (two hours of sleep) elevated levels of pro-inflammatory immune cytokines, as well as cortisol and epinephrine (stress hormones), and napping restored them to pre-deprivation levels. Another study found that two hours of sleep elevated immune cell levels while a thirty-minute nap followed by an eight-hour sleep the following night restored them back to normal.

Aside from sleep deprivation, inflammation also triggers daytime sleepiness and napping. Those with chronic inflammatory conditions nap much more frequently. This seems logical given sleep's anti-inflammatory effects, however it has little effect when severe inflammation such as chronic inflammation is involved.

A few variables influence napping's effectiveness:

1. **Nap purpose.** Biological effects are determined by the reason you nap, such as due to sleep deprivation, in preparation for sleep loss, in response to inflammation, or for pleasure.

2. **Nap duration.** Short naps (<ten minutes) help you feel alert immediately but effects deteriorate within a couple of hours. Longer naps (30–60 minutes) trigger grogginess on waking but alertness lasts much longer.

3. **Nap timing.** Late naps within 5–6 hours of bedtime are detrimental to nighttime sleep. Optimal nap time is about 7.5 hours after waking, so between 1 p.m. and 3 p.m. for most people.

For optimal benefits without grogginess take a 10–20 minute nap between 1 p.m. and 3 p.m.

EAT MORE FRUITS AND VEGETABLES

You won't find a more important food group for your immune health than fruits and vegetables. Here are the five main reasons why:

1. **Vitamins and minerals.** Nutrients important for immunity, such as vitamins A, C, D, and E and minerals zinc, iron, and selenium, are abundant in fruits and vegetables, particularly vegetables.

2. **Phytonutrients.** Phytonutrients such as polyphenols are probably the number one reason to eat lots of fruits and vegetables. They provide antioxidant, anti-inflammatory, detoxification, microbiota, and blood sugar–regulating benefits, and studies prove that they help many immune-related conditions.

3. **Prebiotics.** Fruits and vegetables provide important prebiotics (e.g., fiber and oligosaccharides) that support the development of a healthy microbiota, which is a requirement of strong immune health. They also contain compounds such as polyphenols that strengthen the microbiota. If organic and purchased from quality sources they can also be a useful source of healthy bacteria and other microorganisms.

4. **Acid balance.** Fruits and vegetables raise the pH of your blood, making them your main weapon against an otherwise overly acidic diet (meat, fish, grains, dairy, and processed foods, which lower pH), which is linked to inflammation, immune impairment, and other health problems.

5. **A lower calorie diet.** Consuming lots of vegetables is a healthy way of eating lots of food without consuming excessive amounts of calories (starchy vegetables aside). One of the main reasons behind excess body fat, which is proven to impair immune function, is an excessive calorie intake, largely caused by consuming

lots of calorie-dense foods such as processed foods, animal products, and grains. Increasing vegetable intake means eating less of these foods without going hungry.

A serving of fruits and vegetables is defined as 80 grams, which is the equivalent to one apple or 3 heaped tablespoons of a vegetable. Aim for 800 (or more) grams a day, or ten servings.

In general, vegetables are more nutritionally rich and should provide the majority of your intake. However, many people prefer fruits as they are sweeter. This is usually because the prevalence of sugar in the diet has biased their palate and gut microbiota toward sweet, rather than bitter, foods. Luckily, by gradually introducing more vegetables, you can change your palate over time.

Of the vegetables, mushrooms, cruciferous vegetables, and allium vegetables are the richest sources of immune-boosting nutrients, while berries are the richest fruits.

ENJOY FERMENTED FOODS

Fermented foods have made a comeback in recent years, and that's great news for your immune system. Fermentation is the breakdown of sugars and fibers by bacteria and yeast. Its original purpose was for food preservation, but in the modern era it's primarily used to improve gut microbiota health, though benefits extend beyond this.

There are a number of immune benefits associated with fermented foods, including:

- Increased nutritional content—especially nutrients important for immune health, including vitamin C, vitamin K, zinc, and phytonutrients (polyphenols)
- Repopulating and feeding the gut microbiota with new and existing strains, which aids digestion and immunity
- Lowering inflammation and stimulating the anti-inflammatory benefits of gut bacteria
- Stimulating immune response (natural killer cells)
- Reduced duration of the common cold
- Providing antioxidant, detoxification, and antimicrobial benefits
- Combating respiratory infections and digestive problems (e.g., irritable bowel syndrome)
- Increased insulin resistance
- Improving inflammatory-related conditions including depression and anxiety, diabetes, allergies, asthma, metabolic syndrome
- Lowering total cholesterol and low-density lipoprotein levels

The benefits of fermented food vary depending on the food and fermentation process used. Check online to identify which foods are best suited to your needs. However, using a variety of fermented foods will provide the greatest mix of benefits.

Fermented foods that are good for your immune health include kefir, sauerkraut, tempeh, natto, kombucha, miso, kimchi, yogurt, and sourdough bread.

Many fermented foods can also be made at home, which is surprisingly simple and allows you to have complete control over the ingredients used. If you'd rather skip right to eating, you can purchase different fermented options at health stores. Just be careful of unwanted ingredients such as sugar, artificial preservatives, and other food chemicals.

POLLINATE YOUR IMMUNE SYSTEM

Bee pollen has been consumed for thousands of years for its huge array of health benefits—many of which are linked to the immune system. It contains over 250 compounds that can benefit your health, including proteins, fats, carbohydrates, vitamins, minerals, phytonutrients, enzymes, and coenzymes. Its immune benefits include:

1. **Anti-inflammatory.** Bee pollen contains several compounds that have anti-inflammatory effects on the body.
2. **Antioxidants.** Compounds in bee pollen strengthen your internal antioxidant system or have specific antioxidant properties such as flavonoids and carotenoids.
3. **Antimicrobial.** Bee pollen contains antimicrobial compounds that can kill harmful bacteria (e.g., E. coli, salmonella, and Pseudomonas aeruginosa).
4. **Wound healing.** Bee pollen extracts applied to a burn wound can accelerate healing.
5. **Anti-allergy.** Bee pollen can reduce the severity and onset of allergies by inhibiting the function of mast cells, which play important roles in the early and late phases of an allergic reaction.

The quality and properties of bee pollen vary greatly from product to product. Properties of the pollen change depending on the flowers used and breed of bee. Some pollen products are low quality and high in heavy metals. In order to ensure you have the highest quality, freshest, and most beneficial pollens from healthy bees, look for pollens from local, trusted, ethical producers. Anyone known to react to bee products or bee stings should avoid consuming bee pollen.

You can take bee pollen in the form of granules added to smoothies or yogurt, or in a capsule as a supplement.

EAT MORE RAW FOODS

When you cook food you don't just affect the temperature, taste, look, texture, and smell—you also impact its nutritional profile. Some nutrients are destroyed during cooking, while others become more bioavailable (better absorbed). This has important implications for your immune system. Here are some important things to consider:

1. **Digestion.** Enzymes are lost from food when cooked at temperatures above 117°F, which may reduce digestibility. Some experts argue that these enzymes are not required for digestion; however, they may serve other benefits. Digestibility is improved when cooking foods such as potatoes, legumes, and grains.
2. **Vitamin content.** 50–60 percent of water-soluble vitamins (e.g., vitamin C) are lost during cooking. Vitamin A and minerals are reduced to a lesser extent.
3. **Bioavailable antioxidants.** Some antioxidants become more bioavailable when heated (e.g., lycopene and beta-carotene).
4. **Microbe content.** Both harmful and beneficial microbes are killed when cooked above 140°F.
5. **Mineral absorption.** Phytates (which block mineral absorption) are destroyed when cooking legumes and grains.

Eating a combination of cooked and raw foods appears to be best for all-around nutritional and immune benefits, however the typical Western diet is heavily centered around cooked foods, neglecting raw foods and their benefits.

Aside from eating raw nuts, seeds, vegetables, and fruits, you can introduce more raw foods into your diet through raw dairy produce, as well as fermented and sprouted foods. Also avoid cooking at high temperatures. Instead, try to use lighter cooking methods such as steaming and stir-frying, and reduce cooking times.

UNCOVER GENETIC MUTATIONS

Your genetics have a huge influence on your biology and health—but they don't define it. This is because each cell only expresses a fraction of its genetic code at any point in time. Science has taught us that it's the environment of the gene/cell that determines which genes are active or not. Your lifestyle, environment, emotions, and other factors determine this environment. Aside from this, your health is altered when your genetic code changes.

Genetic changes, or "mutations," can arise from copying errors that occur when your cells divide to make new cells. These are called single nucleotide polymorphisms (SNPs). Every gene consists of sequences of the nitrogenous bases adenine, guanine, cytosine, and thymine, which code for the amino acids that shape biological function. DNA sequences can be thousands of letters long, and a change in just one letter of this code changes the output, which alters your biology, health, and susceptibility to disease.

SNPs impact everything, including your sleep, digestion, inflammatory processes, and immune function. In fact, a gene doesn't need to be directly involved in the immune system to influence immune health—it just needs to impact an area that influences it (e.g., sleep).

New technology allows us to identify the genetic mutations and any corresponding biological weaknesses. SelfDecode (www.selfdecode.com) offers a great SNP service that includes results, interpretations, and diet, lifestyle, and supplement recommendations that allow you to minimize any weaknesses caused by SNPs.

By identifying your SNPs and making appropriate changes you can make a huge difference to your health and immunity.

ELIMINATE NEGATIVE FOOD REACTIONS

If you eat a food that causes a negative reaction such as a headache, stomach pain, bloating, or rash, there is a strong probability that reaction is immune related.

Food reactions are diverse and can cause virtually any symptom—the most severe being allergies. This is when a food triggers an IgE antibody response that stimulates an aggressive and pretty instant immune cell response that can be life threatening. Milder immune reactions are food sensitivities, also called "hidden food allergies," or "food intolerances." Allergy symptoms are obvious, strong, and pretty instant, while food sensitivity symptoms are mild and can take days to appear, making them harder to spot.

Allergies are usually for life, but fortunately you can heal from food sensitivities. Healing sensitivities is critical to a fully functional, healthy immune system for several reasons. For one thing, if you have a sensitivity to one food you likely have multiple and may not even know it, either because of a lack of symptoms or because of their delayed nature. This is a problem because with many food antigens, every time you eat a meal you will likely trigger an immune response, causing a chronic inflammatory state.

Second, food sensitivities arise when your gut lining is permeable. This means that the junctions between cells that line your gut aren't as tight as they need to be in order to keep harmful invaders out. This leads to partially undigested foods passing through your "porous" gut into the bloodstream. The immune system attacks these "invaders," which causes inflammatory reactions (the food sensitivity symptoms). A leaky gut also leaves you vulnerable to other invaders passing through the gut lining, including harmful microbes and chemical toxins that can cause serious ill health. Leaky gut and food sensitivities are often involved in autoimmune conditions. A tightly sealed gut lining is essential for a healthy immune system.

So how do you heal food sensitivities? This requires:

- Identifying and eliminating food antigens for a short period
- Healing the gut
- Restoring gut microbiota balance
- Addressing the causes of the porous gut such as excessive stress, alcohol, poor diet, exposure to electromagnetic fields, nutritional deficiencies, and more

One of the most accurate methods to detect food sensitivities is the LEAP Mediator Release Test (MRT). The MRT measures changes in the blood from immune mediators that are released during an immune reaction (rather than measuring the immune system's memory, which fails because there can be different types of antibody or immune responses involved). It also overcomes the challenge of asymptomatic or delayed reactions, which methods such as a food diary can never identify.

If you experience food reactions it is important to work with a trained practitioner to test and heal your gut.

USE PROPOLIS FOR ALL-AROUND IMMUNE BENEFITS

Propolis is a product made by bees from tree resin, wax, pollen, and essential oils. It's used as a glue by bees for repairing holes in the hive, but it also has tons of health benefits for us.

Propolis contains over three hundred biologically active compounds, including many with antibacterial, antifungal, antiviral, antiparasitic, antiseptic, anesthetic, and anticancer properties. It is known to provide anti-inflammatory and immune-modulating benefits, and also contains vitamins, minerals, and proteins that aid immunity. Propolis is an especially rich source of polyphenols, which provide its antioxidant and anti-inflammatory benefits. Studies have shown that it helps improve inflammatory diseases including cardiovascular (heart disease and hypertension), neurodegenerative (Alzheimer's), and metabolic (type 2 diabetes) conditions. It's also beneficial for wound healing, oral health, skin conditions, cold sores, and allergies.

Propolis comes in a variety of forms including extracts, tinctures, sprays, dried powder, capsules, syrups, and as a raw resin. You will also find toothpastes, shampoos, skin lotions, and creams that contain propolis. Most research has been done using extracts or tincture forms, with a wide range of dosage being used (50–1,500 milligrams per day). There are no side effects reported, although recent studies show around 4 percent of the world population are allergic to propolis.

Like all other bee products, the effectiveness of propolis depends on its source. Ensure that any propolis you use comes from bee colonies that are not factory farmed or subjected to agricultural chemicals. The properties and benefits of propolis are also influenced by the breed of bee, season, geographical region, and trees used in its production.

GET YOUR PLANT FATS

Plant fats are alpha-linolenic acids (ALAs), an omega-3 fat.

ALA's main biological effects are anti-inflammatory. Supplementing with ALA reduces pro-inflammatory cytokines and c-reactive protein levels, and may improve inflammatory conditions including depression, multiple sclerosis, irritable bowel syndrome, allergies, diabetes, and rheumatoid arthritis. ALA also increases fat burning and, by reducing fat, lowers chronic inflammation levels.

The richest sources of ALA are flax seeds, walnuts, chia seeds, and leafy greens. You can boost ALA intake further by using oils rich in ALA (flaxseed oil, wheat germ oil, walnut oil, etc.). However, these polyunsaturated, fatty acid–rich oils are prone to oxidation, which makes them potentially harmful. It's safer to get ALAs from whole foods. If you do use an ALA plant oil ensure it has been cold pressed and contains antioxidants, and store it in the refrigerator.

ALA can be converted to eicosapentaenoic acid (EPA) and docosahexaenoic acid (DHA), which are essential to health and immunity. However, conversion rates are low, and are affected by genetics, age, sex (women convert better) and omega-6 intake. If you are vegan you can support EPA and DHA levels by consuming lots of ALA-rich foods or using algae oil or seaweed oil. (Algae and seaweed are the only plant sources of EPA and DHA.) Algae oils can oxidize, but the benefits of the EPA and DHA outweigh potential harm. Depending on EPA and DHA intake, recommendations for ALA vary between 3 and 12 grams, and 250 milligrams for algae oil.

IMPROVE YOUR WINTER BLUES

Seasonal affective disorder (SAD) affects around 20 percent of the US population every year. Sufferers are usually affected between October and April. SAD symptoms include fatigue, hopelessness, irritability, and loss of interest in social activities.

Although the exact cause is unknown, it's strongly linked to reductions in sunlight duration and intensity during the autumn and winter months. During this period, UVB light (needed for vitamin D and immune health) is virtually nonexistent unless you live close to the equator. Light also regulates the circadian rhythm and provides many beneficial rays beyond UVB, including blue light and red and infrared light, which improve SAD symptoms and immunity.

SAD sufferers have elevated inflammation (pro-inflammatory cytokines), which alongside a vitamin D deficiency contributes significantly to depression. Those suffering from SAD often also suffer from insomnia, eat a poor diet, and exercise less, which only lowers immunity further.

Impaired immunity (including inflammation) and SAD feed into each other. Solutions that address both are most beneficial. These solutions include:

- Getting outdoors when the sun is up as often as possible
- Using a light box or SAD lamp that produces at least 10,000 lux at the distance you plan to use it
- Supplementing with vitamin D3 sulfate
- Experimenting with anti-inflammatory herbs and/or nutrients

Try out these different options to determine which work best for you.

SUPPLEMENT GLUTATHIONE

Glutathione is the most abundant and most important antioxidant in the body. It plays critical roles in health, longevity, and the immune system.

Glutathione is important to your immune system for several reasons. When tissue and cells are exposed to free radical damage (oxidative stress) arising from numerous causes (microbial infections, chemical toxins, heavy metal toxicity, electromagnetic fields, diet, lifestyle, chronic disease, etc.), an inflammatory response is triggered and the immune system is called into action. Glutathione is used to combat the oxidative stress which helps to reduce damage and the inflammatory/immune response. In doing so it reduces the load placed on the immune system. Glutathione also blocks the production of pro-inflammatory cytokines and the NF-kB protein that activates inflammatory genes.

Aside from preventing inflammation, glutathione cleans up the aftermath of an immune response. Some immune cells release free radicals to fight microbes. Glutathione is used to neutralize these free radicals before they cause unnecessary damage.

Elevating glutathione levels improves many immune and inflammatory conditions, including Alzheimer's, depression, anxiety, various lung conditions (including COPD and asthma), heart disease, cancer, diabetes, and autoimmune conditions.

Studies show that supplementing glutathione helps to increase immune response to microbial infection as well as prevent infection. One study supplementing with liposomal glutathione for two weeks produced an increase of 400 percent in natural killer cells and 60 percent in lymphocytes. Supplementing glutathione has an optimal effect when it's used in conditions associated with glutathione deficiency, such as HIV, where it raises immune cell levels (natural killer cells).

Supplementing with standard glutathione is often ineffective as pathways in the liver break it down before it reaches the bloodstream. Instead, supplement glutathione in specialized forms that bypass the liver, such as liposomal glutathione, sublingual (taken under the tongue), inhalation, IV injection, or methyl-glutathione. You can also boost your glutathione levels by supplementing with nutrients/compounds that stimulate and/or support its production or use, including N-acetyl cysteine (NAC), alpha lipoic acid (ALA), selenium, S-adenosyl methionine (SAM-e), and milk thistle. NAC is thought to be most effective, although ALA is another great option.

Supplementing with glutathione may not always be necessary, but should be considered if you are over forty years old (levels drop significantly after this age), glutathione deficient, exposed to high levels of EMF/radiation and/or chemical toxins, have a microbial infection, or require detoxification support.

LET GO OF SHAME

Shame is a powerful emotion that deeply affects your physical and emotional well-being. Research into the immune-related effects of shame has found that it:

- Elevates inflammatory cytokines in proportion to the amount of shame experienced
- Is linked to lower immune function
- Triggers sympathetic nervous system response
- Triggers withdrawal from social interaction
- Can cause permanent impairment to autonomic functioning, leading to chronic anxiety, exhaustion, and depression (when experienced for prolonged periods early in life)

Shame is the sense of feeling worthless. It is often confused with guilt. Shame says, "I am bad," while guilt says, "I did bad." Studies show that shame is much more harmful because it focuses on your identity whereas guilt focuses on behavior. Chronic or toxic shame damages self-esteem, self-acceptance, self-love, and self-worth.

According to top shame researcher Brené Brown, shame is a very harmful emotion because it produces feelings of being unworthy of love and belonging. According to Brown, love and a sense of belonging are strongly tied to our sense of survival. This stems from the need during our early childhood years to be loved by our primary caregivers. After all, without their love our life would be in danger. And a sense of belonging is equally critical as, evolutionarily speaking, being accepted by the tribe was literally a matter of life and death. With these deep survival needs at the root of shame, it's easy to understand why our physiology and immune system respond so strongly to feelings of shame.

The most harmful type of shame is toxic shame, which originates from childhood trauma resulting from abuse. Toxic shame also damages areas of the brain that predispose us to a tendency toward shameful feelings, especially in women. Milder, more frequent shame arises when we experience a threat to our social status or social value. This usually comes up when we fail to live up to societal and cultural standards that we use to define our sense of worth and value.

Common triggers of shame arise in the areas of success, status, career, family, sex, appearance, and material wealth. Becoming aware of these shame triggers in your daily life allows you to interrupt your shame patterns and heal. Brown suggests that the key to overcoming shame is to live wholeheartedly, which encompasses practicing self-compassion, authenticity, resilience, gratitude, joy, intuition, creativity, play, stillness, laughter, song, dance, and meaningful work. Interestingly, these benefit immune health too, proving just how intertwined shame and immune health are. You can begin healing your shame and immune system by developing awareness of your shame triggers and practice living wholeheartedly.

SATISFY YOUR SEX LIFE

It's probably not the first thing that would come to mind when you think about improving your immune health, but there are a number of reasons why sex is beneficial.

One study among college students found that having sex once or twice a week was most effective in lowering infection risks. It produced the optimal response in the immune system located along the protective lining of the gut, respiratory system, reproductive system, and urinary tract. A study of male flies also found that increases in sexual activity (indicated by greater numbers of sexual partners) reduced immune function. These studies suggest that a trade-off may exist between sexual activity and immune function.

In females, frequent sex affects immune cell and antibody levels, which are affected differently depending on where the females are in their menstrual cycle. These changes have not been observed in sexually inactive females. The changes likely occur as the body tries to increase the chance of pregnancy while protecting against infection.

Other factors linked to the immune system include:

- Increased prolactin levels in the body; prolactin improves sleep and is an immune enhancer
- Enhanced immunity via the physical contact, sexual intimacy, and emotional closeness involved, as they increase oxytocin levels and calmness while reducing anxiety and stress hormones
- Increased exchange of microorganisms via physical contact, benefiting the microbiota and immune system
- Lowered inflammation (specifically through kissing)
- A good workout, which benefits immunity

Tap in to your sensual side and boost immunity at the same time!

REDUCE THE EFFECTS OF STRESS

Most people are aware that stress lowers immune health. But how, exactly?

The initial response to stress is the activation of the sympathetic nervous system (SNS) closely followed by stimulation of the HPA axis. The HPA axis is the connection between the hypothalamus, pituitary gland, and adrenal glands. Upon stimulation by the pituitary gland, the adrenal glands release adrenaline and cortisol, the stress hormones.

When the SNS and HPA are activated the immune system produces an inflammatory response. Injury or trauma could be just around the corner, so this response is activated in preparation. All other non-inflammatory pathways and immune cells are inhibited so everything's focused on the emergency. Eventually the delayed effects of cortisol kick in and all immune actions (including inflammation) are stopped.

Excessive or chronic stimulation of the HPA axis is linked to many ill health conditions including digestive problems, damage to the mucosal lining of the gut, obesity, inflammatory conditions, suppressed immune health, and liver impairment. You can help to mitigate some of the harmful effects of HPA stimulation by using adaptogenic herbs, which help the body to react to or recover from physical, mental, or emotional stress. These include:

- Eleuthero (Siberian ginseng)
- Schisandra
- *Rhodiola rosea*
- Cordyceps

These herbs are not just proven adaptogens but are also proven to support immune health. Each of these herbs also have unique properties and benefits so do some research online to find which one is best suited to your needs.

INCREASE YOUR VITAL ENERGY

Western medicine is primarily focused on the physical sciences of biology and biochemistry, but there are other ways of viewing and working with the body that provide powerful health benefits—including those for your immune system.

Researchers such as Wilhem Reich, Claude Swanson, and Nikolai Kozyrev have used science to investigate and demonstrate what ancient traditions have known for centuries: There is a subtle energy that influences our world in powerful ways. Known in the East as "qi" or "chi," and to Reich as "Orgone," this life force, or vital energy, impacts the way your body, mind, and emotions function. Low levels of life force energy are strongly associated with poor physical, mental, or emotional health and disease.

Experiments by Reich in the 1940s and 1950s showed that exposure to life force energy created healing responses within the body that were reflected by measurable changes in the nervous and immune systems as well as "miraculous" recoveries from disease. One such change was a fever-like response (an increase in body temperature) that was thought to indicate an increase in immune function. Experiments by Russian scientists into vital energy have also shown significant improvements in immune function in both animals and humans as indicated by reductions in tumors in mice, as well as increases in T and B lymphocytes (immune cells) and granulocytes (cells that help fight bacterial infection).

There are many ways you can promote better flow of life force energy to aid your immunity and health, including:

- Eating whole natural foods (preferably organic)
- Drinking plenty of clean, filtered water
- Getting out in nature
- Using energy and biofield medicines and therapies
- Using Orgone-based technologies

Energy and biofield medicine/therapy assess and treat the subtle energy fields of the body to help restore the systems (neurological, cardiovascular, respiratory, skeletal, endocrine, emotional, psychological, etc.) back to homeostasis. They include practices like hands-on healing (Reiki, pranic healing, healing touch), homeopathy, magnet therapy, bioelectromagnetic therapies, and electro-dermal therapies.

The flow of life force energy can also be improved by eliminating lifestyle factors that disrupt its flow, including poor diet (processed foods, sugar, alcohol, caffeine, etc.), a sedentary lifestyle, stress, injuries, surgery, emotional stress, dehydration, and pollution/chemical toxins.

INDEX